The *In Practice* Handbooks Series

Series Editors: Margaret Melling and Martin Alder

Current members of *In Practice* Editorial Board

I. D. Baker
A. L. Duncan
J. K. Dunn
H. A. O'Dair
T. J. Phillips
K. A. Urquhart (Chairman)

Titles in print:
Feline Practice
Canine Practice
Equine Practice
Bovine Practice
Sheep and Goat Practice
Swine Practice
Small Animal Practice
Poultry Practice
Canine Practice 2
Equine Practice 2
Bovine Practice 2
Sheep and Goat Practice 2
Feline Practice 2

The *In Practice* Handbooks

Equine
Practice 3

Edited by M. Melling and M. Alder
Editors, *In Practice*

W. B. Saunders

LONDON   PHILADELPHIA   TORONTO   SYDNEY   TOKYO

W. B. Saunders
Company Ltd

24–28 Oval Road
London NW1 7DX

The Curtis Center
Independence Square West
Philadelphia, PA 19106-3399, USA

Harcourt Brace & Company
55 Horner Avenue
Toronto, Ontario M8Z 4X6, Canada

Harcourt Brace & Company, Australia
30–52 Smidmore Street
Marrickville
NSW 2204, Australia

Harcourt Brace & Company Japan
Ichibancho Central Building
22-1 Ichibancho
Chiyoda-ku, Tokyo 102, Japan

A catalogue record for this book is available from the British Library

ISBN 0–7020–2332-9

Typeset by Photo·graphics, Honiton, Devon
Printed and bound in Hong Kong by Dah Hua Printing Press Co., Ltd.

Contents

tests at the surgical facility. Summary

Contributors

E. A. Daniel, University of Liverpool, Department of Veterinary Clinical Science, Leahurst, Neston, Merseyside L64 7TE, UK

G. B. Edwards, University of Liverpool, Department of Veterinary Clinical Science, Leahurst, Neston, Merseyside L64 7TE, UK

S. E. R. Edwards, University of Liverpool, Division of Equine Studies, Leahurst, Neston, Merseyside L64 7TE, UK

G. C. W. England, Royal Veterinary College, Department of Veterinary Surgery, Hawkshead Lane, North Mymms, Hatfield, Hertfordshire AL9 7TA, UK

M. H. Hillyer, University of Bristol, Department of Clinical Veterinary Science, Langford House, Langford, Bristol, Avon BS18 7DU, UK

G. M. Johnston, West End Cottage, Upper Green, Higham, Bury St Edmunds, Suffolk IP28 6PA, UK

D. C. Knottenbelt, University of Liverpool, Division of Equine Studies, Department of Veterinary Clinical Studies, Leahurst, Neston, Merseyside L64 7TE, UK

T. S. Mair, Bell Equine Veterinary Clinic, Butchers Lane, Mereworth, Maidstone, Kent ME18 5QA, UK

B. C. McGorum, Royal (Dick) School of Veterinary Studies, Department of Veterinary Clinical Studies, Veterinary Field Station, Easter Bush, Roslin, Midlothian EH25 9RG, UK

M. C. A. Schramme, Royal Veterinary College, Department of Farm Animal and Equine Medicine and Surgery, Hawkshead Lane, North Mymms, Hatfield, Hertfordshire AL9 7TA, UK

C. H. C. Thursby-Pelham, Bushy Farm Veterinary Clinic, Breadstone, Berkeley, Gloucestershire GL13 9HG, UK

E. D. Watson, Royal (Dick) School of Veterinary Studies, Department of Veterinary Clinical Studies, Veterinary Field Station, Easter Bush, Roslin, Midlothian EH25 9RG, UK

Foreword

The importance of continuing professional development for the veterinarian has reinforced the value of the articles presented in *In Practice*. Originally published as a clinical supplement to *The Veterinary Record*, *In Practice* is now firmly established as a prime source of information for the experienced veterinary clinician and student. The articles, each specially commissioned from acknowledged authorities on their subject, are selected by an editorial board representing a broad spectrum of veterinary expertise with the aim of updating existing information or introducing new developments leading to changes in practice.

The convention of casting the articles in the form of 'opinionated reviews' with the emphasis, where appropriate, on differential diagnosis has proved extremely successful and continues to be a distinguishing feature of *In Practice*.

Republishing selected articles, each updated by the author, as *In Practice Handbooks* has proved very popular. For ease of reference, each handbook deals with a particular species or group of related animals. The present volume is one of the third series in what is likely to be a continuing set of *In Practice Handbook* titles.

CHAPTER 1

Euthanasia of Horses – Alternatives to the Bullet

DEREK KNOTTENBELT

Euthanasia of horses is probably one of the most demanding procedures a veterinary surgeon is likely to face. There are emotive issues involved which make it akin to the euthanasia of small animals and logistics which make it akin to the euthanasia of farm animals. The safety of personnel in the vicinity is paramount and adequate restraint and facilities are vitally important. Notwithstanding these requisites, veterinary surgeons are bound to find themselves in the position of having to compromise, and a working knowledge and experience of different techniques is, therefore, useful. The disposal of carcases is also an important consideration but it should in no way be allowed to take precedence over the welfare of the animal or the skill of the operator. If euthanasia is elective, then arrangements should be made in advance (with a knacker, hunt kennels, etc.) for immediate carcase disposal.

CHOOSING THE SITE

In an emergency the site chosen for euthanasia is often predetermined. Elective euthanasia, however, should only be performed after carefully assessing the environment to ensure safety and efficiency. The ease of access for the knacker wagon should be considered, as should the possibility of the horse's fall creating additional difficulties. Euthanasia alongside a previously-prepared grave is fraught with danger; euthanasia in a loose box can also be very dangerous for all parties.

THE ALTERNATIVES

Death is said to have occurred when all reflex activity has ceased and both respiration and heart function have stopped (the heart may beat for up to 20 minutes following shooting). In considering alternatives to the use of a free bullet firearm, it is important to realize that this method does have obvious advantages when used by experienced veterinary surgeons (i.e. speed, carcase disposal and cost). The major disadvantages are also obvious (danger to personnel, the requirement for experience and a firearms licence). Moreover, it is aesthetically displeasing to the public, although most recognize it as the accepted method. The ideal euthanasia technique would have the properties summarized in Table 1.1.

Three alternative techniques are discussed below – pentobarbitone injection (with or without a premedicant), thiopentone sodium injection with pentobarbitone (with or without a premedicant muscle relaxant and/or sedative), and quinalbarbitone sodium and cinchocaine hydrochloride injection (with or without a premedicant). It should be noted that severance of the aorta per rectum, although often reported, is a very difficult procedure. It is not without danger to the veterinary surgeon, nor is it painless for the horse. Furthermore, death is slower and more violent than is commonly reported. This technique should therefore not be undertaken lightly.

Table 1.1 Properties of the ideal agent/method of euthanasia.

Death should be quiet and instantaneous without any premonition

The agent should be safe for the operator and the public

The agent should be easily handled and stored

The agent should be convenient to administer

There should be no problem with carcase utilization

PENTOBARBITONE INJECTION

Prerequisites

(1)   A suitable volume (calculated at 1 ml per 3 kg bodyweight) of 200 mg/ml pentobarbitone sodium preloaded into the minimum number of syringes.
(2)   A suitable premedicant, preferably an alpha$_2$-agonist at full sedative dose.
(3)   A previously placed 14 gauge (G) jugular catheter.
(4)   Suitable restraint and choice of site (see above).

Method

The horse is restrained and the jugular catheter placed. The premedicant is administered by slow intravenous injection via the catheter and time is allowed for it to exert its maximal effect. The pentobarbitone is then administered as fast as possible; it should be noted that large syringes are better but may be difficult to handle.

The horse will collapse after 30–40 seconds (longer if premedicated), with death occurring within 3 minutes of collapse. Some gasping and muscular activity may occur and collapse may be violent unless the horse is premedicated.

The advantages and disadvantages of this method are listed in Table 1.2.

Table 1.2 Advantages and disadvantages of pentobarbitone injection.

Advantages	Disadvantages
Quick and readily available	Collapse is violent with agonal gasping unless the horse is heavily premedicated
Cheap	
Non-irritant if accidentally injected extravascularly	Volume of drug required makes the use of several syringes essential, which may be difficult to handle quickly enough
No implications under the Misuse of Drugs Regulations 1985; commercial euthanasia solutions are scheduled so as to preclude the recording of individual usages	Carcase disposal is expensive

THIOPENTONE SODIUM INJECTION WITH PENTOBARBITONE

Prerequisites

(1) Separate preloaded syringes containing 0.1 mg/kg suxamethonium and 10 g thiopentone sodium.
(2) A suitable volume (calculated at 1 ml per 5 kg bodyweight) of 200 mg/ml pentobarbitone sodium preloaded in the minimum number of syringes.
(3) A suitable premedicant, preferably an α_2-agonist, at full sedative dose.
(4) A previously placed 14 G jugular catheter. (Note: this method is unsuitable for 'off the needle' euthanasia.)
(5) Suitable restraint and choice of site.

Method

The horse is restrained and the catheter placed. The premedicant, if required, is administered by slow intravenous injection via the catheter and time is allowed for it to exert its maximal effect. The thiopentone is then administered as a bolus as fast as possible, followed immediately by suxamethonium via the catheter.

Collapse can be expected to occur about 30–40 seconds later, although it may occur after 20–30 seconds if no premedicant is used. The pentobarbitone is then administered as quickly as possible (again, large syringes are preferable but may be difficult to handle). The animal will exhibit muscular fasciculations and trembling with prolapse of the third eyelid. Death usually occurs within 3 minutes of collapse.

The advantages and disadvantages of this method are listed in Table 1.3.

QUINALBARBITONE SODIUM AND CINCHOCAINE HYDROCHLORIDE INJECTION

Prerequisites

(1) A suitable volume (calculated at 1 ml per 15 kg bodyweight) of 400 mg/ml quinalbarbitone sodium with 25 mg/ml

Table 1.3 Advantages and disadvantages of thiopentone sodium injection with pentobarbitone.

Advantages	Disadvantages
Quick	Collapse is violent unless the horse is heavily premedicated, particularly so in excited horses
Easily understood method with similarities to anaesthetic induction	
	Complicated procedure involving numerous syringes and injections
No implications under the Misuse of Drugs Regulations 1985, as the drugs are suitably scheduled for use in practice without the need to record individual usages	The volume of drug required makes the use of several syringes essential, which are difficult to handle quickly enough
	Muscular spasms and trembling may be aesthetically displeasing
	Carcase disposal is expensive

cinchocaine hydrochloride (Somulose, Arnolds) preloaded into a single syringe. A dose of 25 ml for horses under 145 cm (14.2 hands) in height and 50 ml for larger horses has been recommended (Knottenbelt *et al.*, 1994).

(2)   A suitable premedicant, such as an α_2-agonist, at full sedative dose. Xylazine should not be used as a sedative prior to the administration of a quinalbarbitone and cinchocaine combination as excitement may be induced and death delayed.

(3)   A previously placed 14 G jugular catheter.

(4)   Suitable restraint and choice of site.

Method

The horse is restrained and the jugular catheter placed. The selected premedicant is administered by slow intravenous injection and time is allowed for it to exert its maximal effect. The full dose of the quinalbarbitone sodium and cinchocaine hydrochloride mixture is then administered over 12–15 seconds. The horse is restrained by keeping its head down and allowed to collapse gently. Collapse can be expected about 30–40 seconds after the start of the injection; if a premedicant is used it will be delayed to 40–50 seconds. There may be an occasional gasp for up to 2 minutes after collapse; death usually occurs within 3 minutes of collapse.

The advantages and disadvantages of this method are listed in Table 1.4.

CHOICE OF METHOD

The author recommends the use of quinalbarbitone and cinchocaine as an alternative to the free bullet firearm for euthanasia

Table 1.4 Advantages and disadvantages of quinalbarbitone sodium and cinchocaine hydrochloride injection.

Advantages	Disadvantages
Quick	Premedication with xylazine is contraindicated
Wide dose range makes accurate dosage unnecessary	Solution is viscous making the required speed of injection potentially difficult to control (a catheter of minimum 14 G should be used)
Relatively cheap	
Single injection syringe contains the total volume of the drug combination	
	Carcase disposal complications (expensive)
Non-irritant if accidentally injected extravascularly	Drug combination is classified as Schedule 2 under the Misuse of Drugs Regulations 1985, requiring that acquisitions/usages be recorded in a register
Collapse predictable even in excited or exhausted horses	
	Too rapid an injection causes an unacceptably violent and prolonged period to death (horse effectively dies of heart failure)
	Slow injections induce 'normal' collapse but a prolonged death (horse is effectively anaesthetized)
	Occasional mild muscular trembling in upper forelimb and gasping

of horses. The method is safe and convenient and is least likely to be associated with complications and aesthetically unacceptable effects. It is nonetheless very important to counsel all attendants carefully as to the possible untoward effects before the procedure is performed. Carcase disposal considerations should not be the primary concern of the veterinary surgeon called upon to perform euthanasia. His or her responsibilities are first and foremost the welfare of the animal and the safety of the attendants.

REFERENCES AND FURTHER READING

American Veterinary Medical Association Panel on Euthanasia (1986) *Journal of the American Veterinary Medical Association* **188**, 252–268.
Jones, R. S. (1993) Euthanasia of horses. *Equine Veterinary Education* **4**, 154–157.
Jones, R. S. (1993) Euthanasia in horses. *RCVS Newsletter*, February, London, Royal College of Veterinary Surgeons.
Knottenbelt, D. C., Jones, R. S., Brazil, T. J., Proudman, C. J., Edwards, S. R. & Harrison, L. J. (1994) Humane destruction of horses with a mixture of quinalbarbitone and cinchocaine. *Veterinary Record* **134**, 319–324.

CHAPTER 2

Artificial Insemination

ELAINE WATSON

The uptake and widespread acceptance of artificial insemination (AI) in horses has lagged behind that in other species. Most breed societies will now allow registration of progeny conceived by AI, but thoroughbreds produced by AI cannot be registered with Weatherbys. It is important that veterinary surgeons can perform these techniques successfully rather than allow lay personnel to offer what may be a less than adequate service to horse breeders.

MANAGEMENT OF THE STALLION

ASSESSMENT OF BREEDING SOUNDNESS

Before a stallion is accepted into an artificial insemination programme, a thorough examination for breeding soundness should be performed. Evaluation of the stallion should include:

(1) History.
(2) General physical examination.
(3) Examination of the external genital organs.
(4) Evaluation of libido.

(5) Evaluation of two semen samples collected 1 hour apart (see below).
(6) Bacteriological culture of swabs from the urethra, urethral fossa and penile sheath for venereal pathogens including *Taylorella equigenitalis*.
(7) Confirmation that the stallion is seronegative for equine viral arteritis or, if vaccinated, was seronegative prior to vaccination.

SEMEN COLLECTION

The commonest method of collecting semen is with an artificial vagina. It is important that this is either fitted with a disposable plastic liner which is changed between stallions or that the rubber liner is thoroughly cleansed between stallions. The best way to clean the rubber liner is to wash it with non-residual soap, rinse well, dry, and then to soak it for 30 minutes in 70% alcohol before hanging it up to dry. To ensure that there are no traces of alcohol left on the rubber it is advisable to rinse the liner with sterile saline and dry thoroughly before use.

Immediately before semen collection, the artificial vagina is filled with water to attain an internal temperature of 45–50 °C. It is important that adequate pressure is exerted on the horse's penis and, therefore, it is usually better to overfill the artificial vagina and then let some water out after assessing the size of the stallion's erect penis. Sterile, water-soluble, non-spermicidal lubricating jelly, such as K-Y Jelly (Johnson & Johnson), should be applied with a clean plastic sleeve to the top two-thirds of the artificial vagina. Because the lubricant dries out quickly it is advisable to leave the sleeve in place until just before collection. The sleeve will also reduce heat loss and prevent contamination.

The stallion should be teased with an oestrous mare until he achieves a full erection. The penis is then rinsed with warm water (42 °C) and dried with soft paper towels (water kills sperm); the person washing and collecting semen from the stallion should wear long plastic disposable gloves to avoid passing infection from one stallion to another (Fig. 2.1). A jump-mare is then positioned and restrained with a twitch. With the collector standing on the stallion's left side slightly behind the stallion handler and holding the artificial vagina in his or her left hand,

(A)

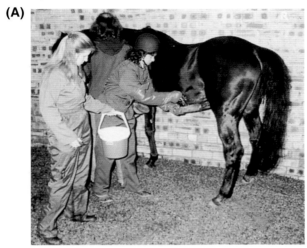

(B)

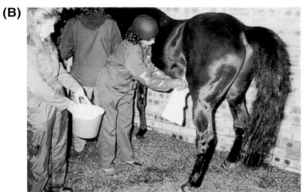

Fig. 2.1 The stallion's erect penis is rinsed with clean, warm water (A) and dried thoroughly (B) before semen collection.

the stallion is allowed to mount the mare. The penis is guided into the artificial vagina which is placed at an angle comfortable for the stallion (Fig. 2.2). The collector's right hand should be placed at the base of the penis to detect ejaculatory pulses. After ejaculation, the anterior end of the artificial vagina is lowered gradually until it is almost vertical as the stallion slides off the mare. The semen should be collected into an insulated receptacle which is non-spermicidal; a Whirl-Pak bag (Astell Hearson, London) or a baby's bottle may be used (Fig. 2.3).

If semen is to be collected regularly from a stallion, he can be taught to use a phantom mare.

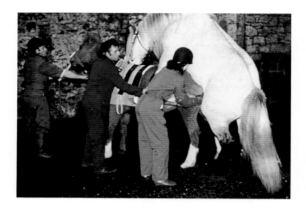

Fig. 2.2 The stallion's penis is guided into the artificial vagina by the collector. It is advisable for the collector to wear a hard hat.

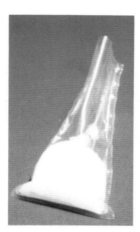

Fig. 2.3 Extended semen in Whirl-Pak bags; the metal tops have been removed from the bags to avoid puncturing the plastic. The air should always be evacuated from the bag before closing it with a rubber band. Two bags should be used as the inner one frequently leaks!

Preparation of the jump-mare

The jump-mare should be docile and can either be a mare in oestrous or an oestrogen-treated ovariectomized mare. She should be swabbed as described by the Horserace Betting Levy Board (1997) to ensure that she is clear of contagious equine metritis and other venereally transmitted bacterial diseases.

The mare's tail should be bandaged or placed inside a plastic sleeve. The perineal region and flanks of the mare should be washed between stallions or a blanket placed over her hindquarters and changed between stallions. Disposable gloves should be worn when washing the mare.

Semen evaluation

Semen evaluation should include assessment of the following.

Gross appearance

Volume

Motility

To estimate motility a drop of semen is placed on a microscope slide, covered with a clean coverslip and put on a warm (38 °C) microscope stage. Motility is observed at ×200 magnification. The percentage of motile sperm (total motility) and percentage progressing forward and rotating (progressive motility) should be recorded.

pH

The pH should be 7.2 to 7.6. If higher, check for contamination with urine or disinfectants. Infection in the genital tract can also raise the pH of semen.

Concentration

Concentration ($\times 10^6$/ml) is measured using a haemocytometer or a calibrated spectrophotometer.

Total number of sperm

The total number of sperm ($\times 10^9$) = volume × concentration.

Morphology

Total number of usable sperm

The total number of usable sperm ($\times 10^9$) = total number of sperm $\times$ % progressively motile $\times$ % morphologically normal. There should be at least 1 billion in the second ejaculate and approximately twice that number in the first ejaculate.

Longevity of motility

This should be assessed in both raw and extended semen at 4 °C and 22 °C in dark, airtight containers. Longevity of motility at 4 °C is important in stallions being used in a chilled transported semen programme, and at 22 °C in stallions where semen is being used on the day of collection. Semen from some stallions loses motility rapidly on storage. Semen from individual stallions responds differently to extender combinations. It is important, therefore, to check a range of extenders and antibiotics and choose the combination which results in the best longevity of motility. In some stallions, longevity of motility can be markedly improved by removing the seminal plasma by centrifugation and resuspending in semen extender.

Toleration to freezing

If semen from a stallion is to be frozen, a test freeze must be performed to evaluate how well sperm from that particular stallion tolerate the freezing process. Before a stallion is accepted for use in an AI programme it is also important that successful test inseminations are achieved with the preserved semen.

Semen handling and evaluation

With some models of artificial vagina it is possible to incorporate a semen filter to retain the gel fraction so that the collected semen is ready for immediate evaluation (Fig. 2.4). Using this method fewer sperm are lost as they do not mix with the gel. If the semen has not been filtered during collection, it should be filtered as soon as possible after collection. All equipment coming into contact with the semen should be pre-warmed to 38 °C.

The following measurements should be recorded:

(1) Volume.
(2) Concentration ($\times 10^6$/ml in gel-free fraction).
(3) Total and progressive motility.
(4) Total number of progressively motile sperm (volume $\times$ concentration $\times$ % progressively motile).
(5) Sperm morphology; this should be checked at the start of the breeding season and at intervals thereafter.

As soon as this preliminary assessment has been performed the semen should be diluted with an equal volume of semen extender (seminal plasma is detrimental to sperm survival) (Table 2.1).

If semen is to be used fresh, it should be allowed to cool to room temperature (22 °C) and maintained in a dark, airtight atmosphere. It should normally be used within 4 hours of collection; pregnancy rates are likely to be inversely proportional to the length of time the semen is left after collection. If the semen is to be transported and chilled it should be diluted with at least two parts (but usually four or eight parts) extender containing antibiotic. If possible, the semen should be diluted to 50 million sperm/ml as semen longevity appears to be optimal at this concentration. Although the recommended minimum insemination dose for a mare is 300 million progressively motile

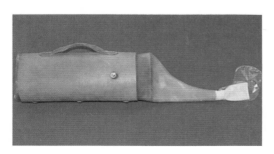

Fig. 2.4 Artificial vagina (Missouri model) with a semen filter incorporated into the collection bag.

Table 2.1 Semen extenders for artificial insemination.

(1)	Instant non-fat dry milk	2.4 g
	Glucose	4.9 g
	Penicillin, crystalline	150 000 U
	Dihydrostreptomycin, crystalline	150 000 μg
	Make up to 100 ml with sterile distilled water	
(2)	Instant non-fat dry milk	2.4 g
	Glucose	4.9 g
	Sodium bicarbonate (7.5%)	2.0 ml
	Gentamicin sulphate (reagent grade: 50 mg/ml)	100 mg
	Add the sodium bicarbonate to the milk or gentamicin before adding the gentamicin to the extender. Make up to 100 ml with sterile distilled water	
(3)	Instant non-fat dry milk	2.4 g
	Glucose	4.9 g
	Ticarcillin	100 mg
	Make up to 100 ml with sterile distilled water	

sperm, it is usual to send approximately one billion progressively motile sperm per insemination dose of 20 ml.

There are two accepted methods of chilling semen. One is to place the semen in an Equitainer (Hamilton-Thorne Research, South Hamilton, Mass, USA), which will maintain it at 4–6 °C for up to 72 hours provided the container is not opened (Fig. 2.5). Similar cooling rates can be achieved by placing the packaged semen in a 15 cm diameter container filled with 500 ml water at 37 °C. The container is then refrigerated at 5 °C. If the latter technique is used the cooled semen can be transported in an insulated flask containing iced water.

It is usual to send two doses of semen so that a mare can be inseminated on two consecutive days. However, in the author's opinion it is preferable to inseminate all the semen upon receipt rather than leaving a dose in the Equitainer. It is important that a sample is retained at the stud farm to record the sperm motility every 24 hours.

If the semen is to be frozen a variety of techniques can be used. High sperm numbers are required and therefore either only the sperm-rich fraction of semen is collected or the semen is concentrated by centrifugation. The sperm are suspended in a special freezing extender and then chilled and frozen in 0.25 or 0.5 ml straws.

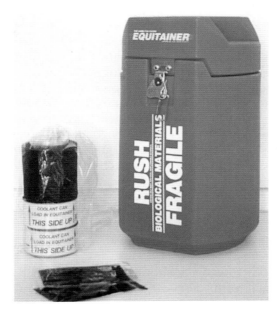

Fig. 2.5 Equitainer with contents displayed. The Equitainer is first loaded with the two coolant cans which should have been placed in a deep freeze for at least 24 hours before use. The semen is packed in the sample cup in the isothermalizer along with the purple ballast bags (pre-warmed to 37 °C). The ballast bags are included to ensure a total volume of between 120 ml and 170 ml; if more than 120 ml of semen is being sent, the bags can be omitted. The sample cup is then closed and the isothermalizer is loaded onto the coolant cans. It is a good idea to place all of the contents into a plastic sleeve before loading them into the Equitainer.

MANAGEMENT OF THE MARE

PRELIMINARY CONSIDERATIONS

Artificial insemination in the mare requires a high degree of veterinary input. Owners should be made aware that AI is not a cheap alternative to natural breeding. Although it is perfectly possible to inseminate a mare at an owner's home, multiple visits will be required. It is far easier if the mare is housed on the practice premises or nearby. The mare need stay only until she ovulates and can then return home. It is also easier if the veterinary surgeon liaises with the stud farm over delivery of semen rather than leaving this to the mare owner. Initial contact between the veterinary surgeon and the stud farm manager should establish semen availability and fertility of the stallion using chilled or frozen semen. The stud farm manager should be given an approximate date for semen shipment. This should be confirmed when the mare comes into oestrus.

The general breeding soundness of the mare should be checked before proceeding with the insemination programme.

For example, it is no use inseminating a mare if she has acute endometritis. In older animals it may be wise to procure an endometrial biopsy to check the degree of chronic irreversible change which occurs in the equine endometrium as a consequence of age. However, detection of pathological processes may not preclude the use of mares in an AI programme. The use of AI can actually increase pregnancy rates in mares which are susceptible to endometritis; because the semen is introduced into the uterus in extender containing antibiotics, bacterial challenge is removed or significantly reduced, decreasing the chances of uterine infection after breeding. Obviously these mares should be cleared of infection prior to AI. Vulvar conformation should be checked with a view to corrective surgery.

INDUCING OVULATION

The stage in the mare's oestrous cycle should be ascertained by the date of the last oestrus (often not available) and by clinical examination of the genital tract. If 6–14 days have elapsed since the last day of oestrus, prostaglandin $PGF_{2\alpha}$ may be administered to bring her into oestrus. Ovulation will occur approximately 10 days later. However, this interval can be highly variable. If, at the time of injection, the mare has a large follicle, ovulation of this follicle may occur before she exhibits signs of oestrus. Furthermore, if the mare had a mid-dioestrous ovulation and if this second corpus luteum is not responsive to $PGF_{2\alpha}$ (i.e. formed less than 6 days previously), the original corpus luteum will lyse but the second will persist and the mare will not exhibit an early return to oestrus.

An alternative method of controlling the time of ovulation is to administer progestogens (e.g. Regumate, Hoechst) in the feed for 10–12 days, giving $PGF_{2\alpha}$ on the last day of treatment. The mare should then return to oestrus and ovulate 7–13 days after the last treatment. It should be borne in mind that it may be difficult to obtain chilled transported semen over weekends, and so treatments should be aimed at inseminating the mare between Tuesday and Saturday, i.e. using semen dispatched on Monday to Friday from the stud farm.

During oestrus, the mare should be teased daily with an unfamiliar gelding or, preferably, a stallion. Serial palpation of the ovaries will monitor growth of the pre-ovulatory follicle.

Ovulation usually occurs on the last or penultimate day of oestrus. Pregnancy rates are highest when the mare is inseminated as close to ovulation as possible, i.e. on the day before ovulation is detected or by 12 hours after ovulation. With frozen semen, insemination should be performed within approximately 6 hours of ovulation; this necessitates ovarian palpation at 12-hourly intervals and inseminating *before and after* detection of ovulation. Alternatively, mares can be examined at intervals of 6–8 hours and inseminated *once* after ovulation is detected. The approach of ovulation is most reliably determined by the presence of a follicle at least 35 mm in size which is palpably softening (Fig. 2.6). At this stage, the intravenous administration of 2500 iu human chorionic gonadotrophin (hCG) will induce ovulation within 24–48 hours in most mares. Repeated administration of hCG over the breeding season may reduce its efficacy. Uterine oedema tends to decrease 1–2 days before ovulation.

INSEMINATION

The mare should be identified using an identity document and prepared for insemination in a clean environment, preferably restrained in stocks. Her tail should be wrapped in a plastic

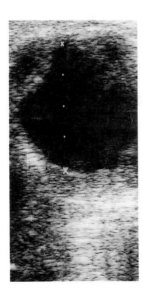

Fig. 2.6 Ultrasound image of a 41 mm pre-ovulatory follicle on the day before ovulation. The follicle is softening and starting to migrate to the ovulation fossa. Note 'pointing' of the follicle.

sleeve or tail bandage and secured out of the way of the perineal region. The mare's rectum should be emptied of faeces to prevent contamination of the area during insemination. The vulva and perineal area should then be cleansed three times with povidone-iodine solution or mild soap (Fig. 2.7). After the final rinse with warm water the area should be dried with clean, soft paper towels (Fig. 2.8).

The semen container should be left unopened until this stage. If a microscope is readily accessible, a drop of the semen should be checked for motility after leaving it on a warm slide for a few minutes; in general, the semen is considered acceptable if the progressive motility is above 30%. The remainder of the semen should be loaded immediately into a sterile plastic syringe without a rubber plunger (do not attach a needle) (Fig. 2.9). The operator should wear a sterile surgeon's glove over a clean rectal sleeve and the arm should be lubricated with a small amount of K-Y Jelly. The sterile insemination pipette should be guided through the cervix with the gloved hand, the syringe then attached and the semen infused into the uterus (Fig. 2.10).

Frozen semen should be thawed according to the stud farm's instructions (usually at 37 °C for 45 seconds). If it has been

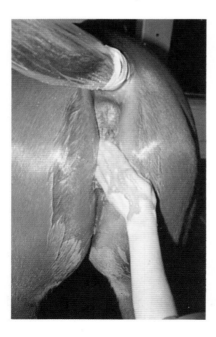

Fig. 2.7 The mare's rectum is cleared of faeces and her vulva and perineal region are washed three times with povidone-iodine solution.

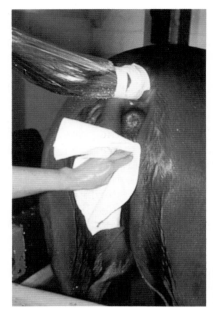

Fig. 2.8 If more than one mare is being inseminated or examined, the operator should wear disposable gloves while washing. After rinsing, the vulva and perineal region are dried with a soft, clean paper towel.

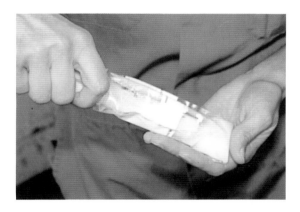

Fig. 2.9 Semen is loaded into an airtight syringe.

imported into the UK it should be accompanied by documentation that the stallion is seronegative for equine arteritis virus. It should then be inseminated as described above.

The mare should be checked for ovulation 12 hours later (where frozen semen is being used), 24 hours later (for chilled semen) or 48 hours later (for fresh semen). It may be necessary

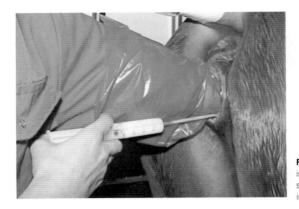

Fig. 2.10 The insemination pipette is guided through the cervix, the syringe attached, and the semen infused into the uterus.

to order another batch of chilled semen if the time of ovulation has been miscalculated. Chilled semen should be used within 48–72 hours of collection.

MONITORING PREGNANCY

Once the mare has ovulated she should be examined by ultra-sonography 16–18 days later to determine whether or not she has a single normal embryonic vesicle (Fig. 2.11). Particular

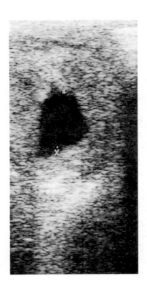

Fig. 2.11 Seventeen-day-old embryonic vesicle.

attention must be paid to the number of embryos if the mare had a double ovulation. If she is pregnant, further examinations should be performed at around 30, 42 and 63 days after ovulation to monitor the development of the conceptus.

If the mare is not pregnant and there is no clinical evidence of any genital abnormalities, she should be reinseminated at the next oestrus. In either case the stud farm manager should be informed of the outcome.

ADVANTAGES AND DISADVANTAGES OF AI

The advantages of AI in the horse include:

(1) Disease control.
(2) Reduces the possibility of traumatic injury to a valuable mare or stallion.
(3) Allows use of stallions or mares with poor breeding habits or injuries.
(4) Provides a constant monitor of semen quality.
(5) Avoids overuse of a stallion and allows several mares to be bred on the same day.
(6) Can result in higher pregnancy rates than natural service.
(7) Reduces problems of geographic inaccessibility.
(8) Avoids having to transport a mare with a young foal.
(9) Mares and stallions can remain in training.

Disadvantages are:

(1) Often more expensive for the mare's owner owing to the high degree of veterinary involvement.
(2) Mare owners may have to assume a level of responsibility for the management of the mare.
(3) Repeat inseminations result in increased semen transport costs.

REFERENCES AND FURTHER READING

BEVA Code of Practice for Veterinary Surgeons and Breed Societies in the United Kingdom and Ireland using Artificial Insemination for Breeding Equids. December 1991. BEVA, 5 Finlay Street, London SW6 6HE.

Horserace Betting Levy Board (1997) *Common Codes of Practice for Control of Contagious Equine Metritis and other Bacterial Venereal Diseases and Equine Viral Arteritis*. HBLB, 52 Grosvenor Gardens, London SW1W 0AU.

Pickett, T. B. W., Squires, E. L. & McKinnon, A. O. (1987) *Procedures for collection, evaluation and utilization of stallion semen for artificial insemination*. Colorado State University, Animal Reproduction Bulletin Number 03.

CHAPTER 3

Real-time Ultrasonography for the Diagnosis and Management of Equine Pregnancy

GARY ENGLAND

The use of diagnostic real-time B-mode ultrasound for medical imaging has increased considerably over the past 15 years. Ultrasonography has had a particular impact upon the field of veterinary reproduction where it has proved valuable as both a clinical and a research tool.

PRINCIPLES OF DIAGNOSTIC ULTRASOUND

Diagnostic ultrasound utilizes sound frequencies between 2 MHz and 10 MHz which are above the audible range. Ultrasound is produced by the application of a voltage to piezo-electric crystals causing them to change in size, thereby producing a pressure or ultrasound wave. Returning echoes deform the same crystals which generate a surface voltage. These voltages are displayed on an oscilloscope. In the case of brightness modulation (B-mode) ultrasonography, the returning echoes are displayed as dots, the brightness of which is proportional to their amplitude. Real-time B-mode ultrasound is a dynamic imaging system where information is continually updated and displayed on a monitor.

In any given tissue, attenuation of ultrasound is related to its wavelength, the density of the tissue, the heterogeneity of the tissue and the number and type of echo interfaces. In general, ultrasound may be attenuated by reflection, scatter and absorption. For diagnostic ultrasound there is minimal tissue absorption; the greatest proportion of sound is reflected. The amount of reflected sound is proportional to the impedance difference between two tissues. Bright (specular) echoes are produced when a large proportion of the beam is reflected back to the transducer, while non-specular echoes are produced when the beam encounters a structure similar to one wavelength in size. In this case the beam is scattered in many directions and only a small proportion returns to the transducer. These echoes give an organ its characteristic echotexture.

Piezoelectric crystals are arranged together to form an ultrasound transducer, contained within the ultrasound head. The crystals may be arranged in a line (linear array transducer), an arc (sector transducer), mounted upon a rotating wheel (mechanical sector transducer) or arranged in an arc and electronically triggered (phased array transducer). Transducers produce sound of a characteristic frequency. High frequencies allow good resolution although there is greater attenuation of the sound beam in tissues, while low frequencies allow a greater depth of penetration (less attenuation) but with reduced resolution.

EQUIPMENT FOR EXAMINATION OF THE MARE

Linear array transducers are most suited to transrectal imaging because they can be easily held in the hand and manipulated adjacent to the reproductive tract. They allow a large field of view in the near field and are generally robust. Sector transducers may also be used although they are more difficult to manipulate, offer only a small field of view in the near field and are frequently more expensive than linear array transducers.

In an ideal situation, a range of transducers of differing frequencies should be available. For the examination of ovarian structures and of early pregnancy a 7.5 MHz transducer is most suitable, while for the examination of late pregnancy a 3.5 MHz transducer is necessary. A 5.0 MHz transducer offers a compromise which gives a reasonable depth of penetration combined with adequate tissue resolution.

The ultrasound machine should be small and lightweight, have a keyboard to allow identification of the animal and possess electronic callipers to allow measurement of images. Facilities should also be available to record the images. This can be achieved using a thermal printer, a Polaroid camera or a multi-format camera. The thermal printer and Polaroid camera are both portable and produce an immediate hard copy; the former is expensive to purchase although the cost per print is low.

PATIENT PREPARATION

Safety of the operator during the procedure is paramount and, therefore, mares should ideally be restrained in stocks. Foals are best positioned either in front of the stocks or within the stocks adjacent to the mare. Additional restraint may be required for certain individuals; in most cases the application of a twitch is effective.

The mare's rectum should be emptied of faecal material to ensure a good contact between the transducer and the rectal wall. Attempts to manipulate the transducer when the rectum is filled with faecal material may result in tearing of the rectal wall. Should the mare strain during the examination the transducer should be withdrawn. If straining continues it may be necessary to apply a twitch or use a low dose of a sedative agent. The alpha$_2$-agonist drugs are particularly useful for this purpose and are also valuable when the examination is prolonged, for example when attempting to reduce the number of conceptuses. Low doses of detomidine hydrochloride do not appear to interfere with the early developing conceptus.

IMAGING TECHNIQUE

The examination should be performed out of direct sunlight, which can hinder interpretation of images on the ultrasound screen. The ultrasound transducer is usually held within the rectum in the sagittal (longitudinal) plane during imaging. The

G. C. W. *England*

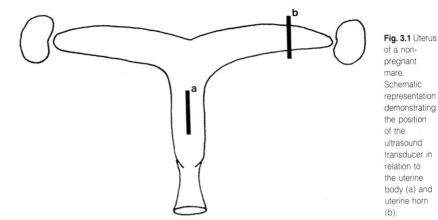

Fig. 3.1 Uterus of a non-pregnant mare. Schematic representation demonstrating the position of the ultrasound transducer in relation to the uterine body (a) and uterine horn (b).

vestibule and vagina lie within the pelvis in the midline. These structures can be imaged with ultrasound but are indistinct. The cervix is located cranial to the vagina, approximately 20 cm cranial to the anal sphincter, and can be identified with ultrasound as a heterogeneous generally hyperechoic region with a rectangular outline. The uterus is roughly 'T' or 'Y' shaped (Fig. 3.1). Therefore, when using a linear ultrasound transducer the outline of the uterine body generally appears rectangular (the transducer is in a sagittal plane); the outline of the uterine horns appears circular (the transducer while orientated in the sagittal plane is positioned in a transverse lane with respect to the uterine horn) (Figs 3.2, 3.3).

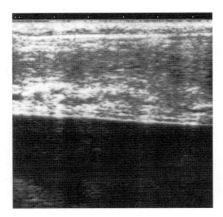

Fig. 3.2 Ultrasound image of the uterine body positioned dorsal to the bladder – sagittal section (7.5 MHz transducer, scale in cm).

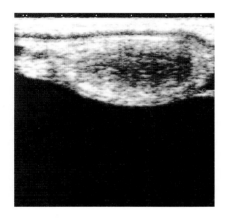

Fig. 3.3 Ultrasound image of the uterine horn positioned dorsal to the bladder – transverse section (7.5 MHz transducer, scale in cm).

The uterus has a central homogeneous, relatively hypoechoic region surrounded by a peripheral hyperechoic layer. The echogenicity of the endometrium and the uterine cross-sectional diameter vary during the oestrous cycle; during oestrus the diameter increases and the uterus becomes increasingly hypoechoic with central radiating hyperechoic lines which are typical of endometrial oedema.

DIAGNOSIS OF PREGNANCY

The use of high-frequency ultrasound transducers allows the early diagnosis of pregnancy in the mare. Clinically, it may be important for pregnancy to be diagnosed before the formation of the endometrial cups and the secretion of equine chorionic gonadotrophin (eCG). This hormone, produced from approximately 40 days to 120 days after ovulation, prevents the mare from breeding despite the absence of a conceptus. Pregnancy should therefore be diagnosed before day 40 if management or termination is likely to be necessary. Examination after day 40 is generally only of value for confirming pregnancy and assessing fetal viability.

EARLY PREGNANCY

The early diagnosis of pregnancy in the mare is highly accurate although there are several potential pitfalls including the confusion of uterine cysts with conceptuses, and the presence of twin conceptuses (see later). The early conceptus can only be imaged when sufficient anechoic yolk sac fluid has been formed. This is usually from 9 days after ovulation, at which time the conceptus appears as a spherical anechoic structure approximately 2 mm in diameter (Fig. 3.4). The dorsal and ventral margins of the conceptus produce characteristic bright specular echoes. Subsequently, the conceptus rapidly increases in size to reach approximately 10 mm in diameter 14 days after ovulation. The outline remains circular (spherical), presumably because of the thick embryonic capsule.

Until day 16 the conceptus is mobile and may be identified either within the uterine horns or the uterine body. This mobile phase is important for the maternal recognition of pregnancy. During pregnancy diagnosis careful attention to imaging of the entire uterus is required – the transducer should be moved slowly from the tip of one uterine horn to the other, and then caudally towards the cervix. From day 17 until day 28 the increase in conceptus diameter is slowed. Transuterine migration usually ceases by day 17. The conceptus becomes fixed in position at the base of one uterine horn, usually the contralateral uterine horn to the previous pregnancy. After fixation, the conceptus rotates so that its thickest portion, the region of the embryonic pole, assumes a ventral position. During this period of orientation the uterine wall adjacent to the dorsal pole of the conceptus becomes thickened. The conceptus generally retains a spherical outline until approximately 18 days after ovulation after which time it may be deformed by pressure from the ultrasound transducer and adjacent viscera. It is not uncommon for the conceptus to appear triangular or flattened in outline.

The embryo may be imaged from approximately 21 days after ovulation, at which time it appears as an oblong hyperechoic structure adjacent to the ventral pole of the conceptus. A heart beat is commonly detected within the embryonic mass from approximately 22 days after ovulation. This appears as a rapidly flickering motion in the central portion of the embryonic mass. From this time onwards the embryo has two poles. Growth of

(A)

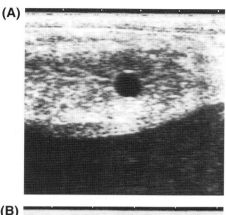

(B)

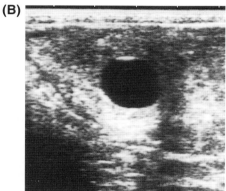

(C)

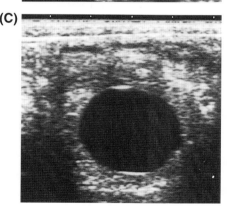

Fig. 3.4 Conceptus 12–22 days after ovulation (7.5 MHz transducer, scale in cm). (A) **Day 12 after ovulation** The anechoic yolk sac is spherical in outline and the conceptus is bordered dorsally and ventrally by characteristic specular echoes. The conceptus is mobile within the uterus. (B) **Day 14 after ovulation** The conceptus is approximately 1 cm in diameter. A region of acoustic enhancement is common ventral to the conceptus. (C) **Day 16 after ovulation** The conceptus has become fixed in the base of one uterine horn. Its outline remains circular (spherical).

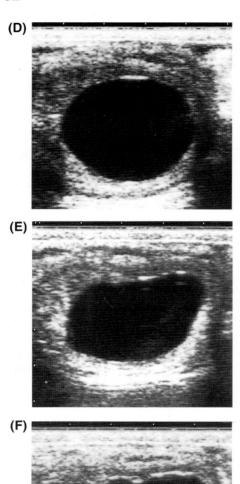

Fig. 3.4 Continued. (D) **Day 18 after ovulation** The conceptus is not spherical and the uterine wall has become thickened, especially dorsally. (E) **Day 20 after ovulation** The conceptus is irregular in outline. The increase in conceptus size is reduced. (F) **Day 22 after ovulation** The embryo (arrow) is imaged adjacent to the ventral margin of the conceptus. A heart beat can be detected at this stage.

the allantois lifts the embryo from the ventral position. The allantois may be identified from day 24, when it appears as an anechoic structure ventral to the embryo (Fig. 3.5). Apposition of the yolk sac and the allantois results in the formation of a curved echogenic line on each side of the embryo. The size of the allantois increases and that of the yolk sac is gradually reduced until, at approximately 30 days afer ovulation, they are similar in volume. At this stage, the echogenic junction between the yolk sac and the allantois is often horizontally directed, although it may be positioned obliquely or vertically.

From day 30 onwards it is possible to image the amnion surrounding the developing embryo. The relatively echogenic amnion is approximately 1 mm thick and is separated from the embryo by a small volume of anechoic amniotic fluid. From this time the diameter of the conceptus again rapidly increases. At 35 days after ovulation the embryo is approximately 15 mm in length and the allantois is three times the volume of the yolk sac.

Continued growth of the allantois and shrinkage of the yolk sac results in the embryo being lifted towards the dorsal aspect of the conceptus and, by days 38 and 40, the fetus is positioned adjacent to the dorsal pole. At day 40, the yolk sac is almost completely absent and the umbilicus which attaches to the dorsal pole can be imaged.

FROM 40 DAYS AFTER OVULATION

Imaging of the pregnancy after the formation of the endometrial cups may be necessary to ensure continued fetal development and assess fetal viability. This may be of value where there is concern about fetal resorption or abortion, or when multiple conceptuses have been managed. The diagnosis of pregnancy with ultrasound at this stage is highly accurate, although in later pregnancy it may be difficult to appreciate fully the presence of multiple conceptuses.

From day 40 after ovulation the yolk sac is collapsed and almost completely obliterated. The umbilicus which incorporates the yolk sac is tortuous and appears relatively hyperechoic (Fig. 3.6). The umbilicus which remains attached to the dorsal pole of the vesicle lengthens, allowing the fetus to move to a ventral position within the conceptus. The fetus is positioned

(A)

(B)

(C)

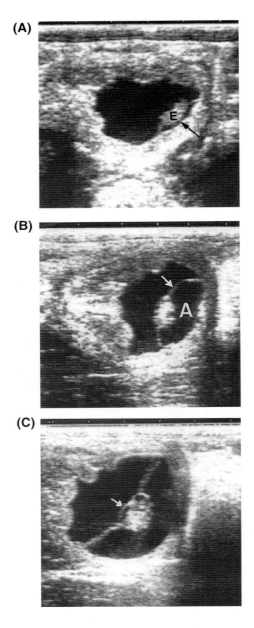

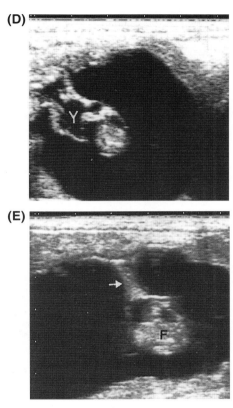

Fig. 3.5 Conceptus 24–40 days after ovulation (7.5 MHz transducer, scale in cm). (A) **Day 24 after ovulation** The embryo (E) is lifted dorsally by the developing allantois (arrow). The yolk sac is irregular in outline. (B) **Day 28 after ovulation** The volume of the allantois (A) is less than that of the yolk sac. The embryo is positioned centrally within the conceptus. Identification of the heart beat is simple at this stage. (C) **Day 32 after ovulation** The allantois exceeds the volume of the yolk sac. The relatively echogenic amnion (arrow) can be imaged surrounding the embryo. (D) **Day 36 after ovulation** The allantois surrounds the yolk sac (Y) and the allantoic membranes are nearly opposed. The amnion is prominent. (E) **Day 40 after ovulation** The yolk sac is almost completely obliterated and the umbilicus can be imaged (arrow). The fetus (F) is several centimetres in length.

(A)

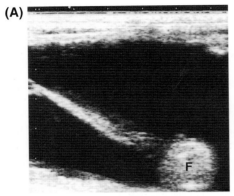

(B)

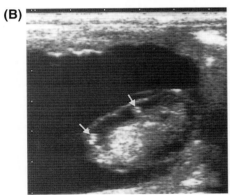

Fig. 3.6 Conceptus from 40 days after ovulation (7.5 MHz transducer, scale in cm). (A) **Day 50 after ovulation** The umbilicus which incorporates the yolk sac has lengthened and the fetus (F) is imaged suspended within the allantois adjacent to the ventral wall of the uterus (transverse image of the fetal abdomen). (B) **Day 60 after ovulation** There is clear differentiation of the fetus. Limb buds can be imaged (arrows) and the amnion can be identified surrounding the fetus.

adjacent to the ventral pole from 50 days after ovulation at which time limb buds can be readily imaged and ballottement of the uterus causes the fetus to float within the allantoic fluid. Fetal movements are commonly seen.

The abdominal and thoracic portions of the fetus can be differentiated after day 50. Pulmonary tissue surrounding the heart is hyerechoic with respect to the liver. The line of separation between the liver and lung (region of the forming diaphragm) can easily be identified. The moving hyperechoic heart valves can be imaged and the great vessels can be traced cranially and caudally. Imaging of the fetal stomach is possible after 55–60 days from ovulation. The stomach is variably filled with anechoic fluid and can be detected caudal to the liver in more than 90% of fetuses from this time onwards.

It has been suggested that fetal sex may be accurately diagnosed 59–68 days after ovulation. Interpretation is difficult and relies upon identifying the position and appearance of the genital tubercle.

It is possible to image fetal eyes from day 60 and measurement of their diameter has been used to estimate the gestational age. Initially, the fetal eye appears as a spherical anechoic structure (Fig. 3.7). From 120 days after ovulation the caudal lens margin can also be identified and later the anterior chamber and ciliary body can be clearly imaged.

The appearance of the fetal skeleton becomes enhanced during late pregnancy; the head, spinal column and ribs produce intense reflections that are easily identifiable. Structures that have been previously described become larger and more easy to image. However, from 150 days onwards it is not always possible to image the entire fetus using high-frequency trans-

(A)

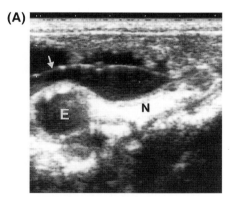

(B)

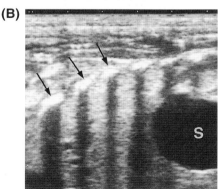

Fig. 3.7 Conceptus during late pregnancy (7.5 MHz transducer, scale in cm). (A) **Day 100 after ovulation** The fetal eye (E) and nasal bones (N) can be clearly identified. The amnion (arrow) surrounds the fetus. (B) **During late pregnancy** The ribs (arrows) cast acoustic shadows and the anechoic fluid-filled stomach (S) can be imaged.

ducers because of their short depth of penetration. The dorsal portion of the fluid-filled uterus can always be imaged and the fetus may be seen by using a lower-frequency transducer either transrectally or transabdominally.

From eight months of pregnancy onwards it may be difficult to image more than a small portion of the fetus because of its large size. Frequently the head can be imaged although ultrasound is reflected by bone, making the image difficult to interpret. In late pregnancy the amniotic cavity is increased in volume and the amniotic fluid contains multiple small echogenic particles.

UTERINE CYSTS

Uterine cysts which originate from either endometrial glandular or lymphatic tissue are not uncommon in the mare. They are characteristically fluid-filled and therefore anechoic, and have a fine, moderately echogenic wall which may not be fully appreciated unless there are multiple cysts or there is free uterine fluid (Fig. 3.8). Cysts may range from several millimetres to several centimetres in diameter. Low numbers of small cysts have no significant effect upon fertility. Larger cysts may be associated with uterine inflammatory disease and may impede the movement of the conceptus.

Uterine cysts may be confused with early conceptuses and, when a conceptus is positioned adjacent to a cyst, these may appear to be twin conceptuses. To avoid these potential problems it is prudent to record the size, shape and position of uterine cysts before breeding.

Cysts may be differentiated from the early conceptus because they:

are often irregular in outline;
may be lobulated;
do not always produce dorsal and ventral pole specular echoes;
do not change position, and change in size only slowly;
frequently are not positioned within the uterine lumen.

In later pregnancy, the presence of an embryo allows the differentiation of a conceptus from a uterine cyst.

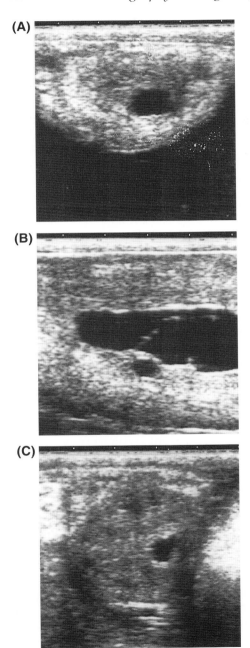

Fig. 3.8 Uterine cysts. (A) Small extraluminal uterine cyst (7.5 MHz transducer, scale in cm). (B) Large extraluminal uterine cysts (5.0 MHz transducer, scale in cm). (C) Small luminal uterine cyst (7.5 MHz transducer, scale in cm).

(D)

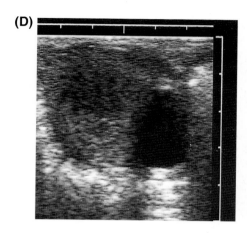

Fig. 3.8 Continued. (D) Multiple large luminal uterine cysts (7.5 MHz transducer, scale in cm).

MULTIPLE CONCEPTUSES

There is great concern over multiple conceptuses in the mare because of their poor prognosis. The primary aim of the clinician is the termination of pregnancy or the reduction of conceptus numbers before the secretion of eCG. Ultrasonography is invaluable in allowing the early diagnosis of multiple conceptuses (Fig. 3.9). The risk of confusion of conceptuses with uterine cysts, as discussed above, should be considered when multiple conceptuses are thought to be present.

Multiple conceptuses may be anticipated when more than one ovulation has been identified, an event which may occur synchronously (from one or both ovaries) or over a period of up to 10 days. The chance of conception with asynchronous ovulations is related to the timing of breeding and the fertility of the stallion.

Conceptuses will vary in size depending upon the ovulation date. Multiple conceptuses are almost always dizygotic, in which case several corpora lutea can be imaged. Multiple conceptuses may be identified adjacent to each other, or in separate positions within the uterine body or horns. Movement of conceptuses occurs independently within the uterus although the pattern of migration is slightly reduced compared with singletons; where conceptus size differs, the smaller conceptus tends to be less motile and remains for longer periods of time within the uterine body.

(A)

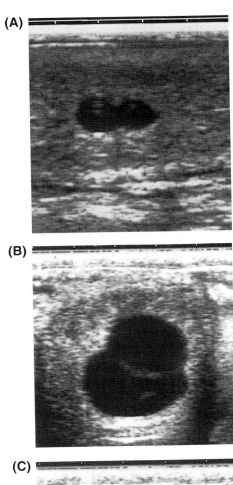

(B)

(C)

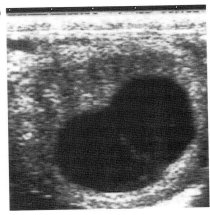

Fig. 3.9 Early multiple conceptuses. (A) Twin conceptuses 13 days after ovulation positioned within the uterine body (5.0 MHz transducer, scale in cm). (B) Twin conceptuses 15 and 16 days after ovulation positioned adjacent to each other in the uterine horn. The small conceptus is compressed into the wall of the larger conceptus (7.5 MHz transducer, scale in cm). (C) Two day 17 conceptuses fixed within the base of the same uterine horn. The line of separation is clearly visible (7.5 MHz transducer, scale in cm).

(D)

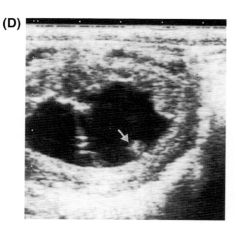

Fig. 3.9 Continued. (D) Two day 22 conceptuses fixed adjacent to each other. Both conceptuses are irregularly marginated; the embryo of one is in the field of view (arrow) (7.5 MHz transducer, scale in cm).

More conceptuses become fixed unilaterally than bilaterally and, therefore, intervention is best planned before day 17 when the conceptus becomes fixed. There is, however, a tendency for natural embryo reduction after day 17 and this appears to be greater for unilateral separate conceptuses. Imaging of bilateral multiple conceptuses and unilateral separate conceptuses is uncomplicated; the diagnosis may be less simple when unilateral multiple conceptuses are adjacently positioned.

During early pregnancy the line of separation between adjacent conceptuses may be difficult to image; however, the conjoined conceptuses may be oblate rather than spherical in outline. Similar problems of diagnosis may also occur when conceptuses are of unequal diameter. Adjacent twin conceptuses may be mistaken for allantoic and yolk sac cavities of a single conceptus of later gestation; the absence of the embryo is, however, diagnostic.

From 21 days to 40 days after ovulation, the diagnosis of most unilateral multiple conceptuses is not difficult. The key to diagnosis is the identification of more than one embryo, Occasionally, one conceptus may be indented by the other, may have an unusually positioned embryo (disorientation) or may have no embryo. These findings are often associated with natural embryonic reduction; however, a similar appearance may also occur with conceptuses of markedly differing ages. After day 50 it may be difficult to image multiple fetuses reliably because of their ventral position within the uterus. The identification of two separate fetuses, each with cardiac movements, is diagnostic and is best achieved using a low-frequency ultrasound transducer.

MANAGEMENT OF MULTIPLE CONCEPTUSES

Multiple conceptuses (frequently twins) should be reduced to a single conceptus or, if possible, the pregnancy terminated before the formation of endometrial cups.

Bilateral twins identified 14 days after ovulation can be managed by manipulating the smaller conceptus towards either the tip of the uterine horn or the cervix, and then crushing it against these structures or the pelvic floor; alternatively, it may be crushed between the fingers and thumb. Following the collapse of the conceptus, the yolk sac fluid disperses throughout the uterus although it may pool at the site of crushing for some time. It is prudent to examine the mare 2 days after the crushing procedure to ensure that the remaining conceptus has continued to develop. Loss of the second conceptus can result from endogenous prostaglandin release.

Unilateral twins identified 14 days after ovulation may be managed in a similar way, although they must first be separated using pressure from the ultrasound transducer. There is no evidence to suggest that anti-inflammatory agents (cyclooxygenase inhibitors) or progestogens protect the remaining conceptus.

When multiple conceptuses are identified from 17 days after ovulation the success rate of selective termination by crushing is reduced. The technique is more difficult to perform for unilateral conceptuses because they will have become fixed and cannot be separated. Following crushing, the released yolk sac and allantoic fluid tend to pool around the remaining conceptus and may be responsible for its subsequent loss. At this later stage of pregnancy the options are to attempt manual crushing of one conceptus risking damage to both, terminate the pregnancy, or allow the pregnancy to continue in the hope that only one embryo will survive; the last option is rarely successful. Repeatedly flattening a conceptus using the ultrasound transducer may sufficiently damage it to produce subsequent loss. Damage is usually characterized by an immediate increase in the echogenicity of the allantoic and/or yolk sac fluid; however, ultrasound examination must be performed 24 hours later to confirm loss of the conceptus.

If multiple conceptuses survive beyond 40 days after ovulation the pregnancy can be monitored until midterm in the hope that one fetus will spontaneously die. It has been suggested that partial starvation of the mare may be successful in reducing the number of conceptuses. Potassium chloride has been injected into the fetal heart under ultrasound guidance and is best performed between 70 days and 110 days after ovulation; this, however, has only been undertaken in a limited number of mares.

EXAMINATION STRATEGY

There are many suggested protocols for the diagnosis and evaluation of pregnancy in the mare. When the time of ovulation is known, a strategy comprising three examinations, performed on days 14, 21 and 35, is suitable in most cases.

FIRST EXAMINATION

The first ultrasound examination should be performed 14 days after ovulation. If a single conceptus is imaged, and there is no suspicion of multiple conceptuses, the mare should be re-examined on day 21.

There may be a suspicion of multiple conceptuses before imaging is performed, however, either because more than one corpus haemorrhagicum was identified or because several large follicles remained after one ovulation and these might have subsequently ovulated. At the time of pregnancy diagnosis, assessment of the number of luteal structures is of value in determining the potential number of conceptuses. Should multiple conceptuses be imaged they may be effectively managed, even if they are adjacently positioned, as they do not become fixed in position until day 17. Imaging early in the mobile phase maximizes the opportunity to eliminate conceptuses manually.

In modern breeding programmes, when mares are mated or inseminated on only one occasion, it is unusual for conceptuses to vary by more than 4 days in age. The identification of a single conceptus at day 14 is therefore likely to be a correct diagnosis. Should this be incorrect and the mare re-examined on day 21, the younger conceptus will be aged 17 days or less, and may still be unfixed and therefore separable from the 21-day conceptus, if necessary. If, on day 14, there is concern over the ability to image a second conceptus (aged 10 or 11 days), because of the presence of endometrial cysts, the availability of only low-frequency ultrasound transducers or operator inexperience, the ultrasound examination should be repeated on day 16.

SECOND EXAMINATION

It is advisable to perform a second ultrasound examination 21 days after ovulation, allowing an assessment to be made of the development of the conceptus. At this stage, the embryo can usually be imaged and the process of orientation evaluated. The identification of a heart beat confirms embryonic viability. Inappropriate development of the conceptus, including abnormal orientation, failure to increase in size and abnormal echogenicity of the yolk sac fluid, is uusually associated with subsequent pregnancy failure.

Examination 21 days after ovulation also enables confirmation that a single conceptus is present and may allow management of multiple conceptuses that were not previously identified.

THIRD EXAMINATION

The third examination should be performed 35 days after ovulation, before the development of endometrial cups and the secretion of eCG. The aim of this examination is to confirm the presence of a normally developed single conceptus. Inappropriate development of the conceptus is best managed by termination of the pregnancy, while multiple conceptuses may be managed by invasive methods.

ABNORMALITIES OF PREGNANCY

The incidence of pregnancy abnormalities in the mare is unknown although there are probably breed and age influences.

The major concerns are embryonic death and fetal death with subsequent abortion. The recognition of any abnormality before the formation of endometrial cups allows intervention which will ensure a return to oestrus.

EMBRYONIC RESORPTION

The greatest incidence of pregnancy loss in the mare occurs before day 25 and the use of diagnostic real-time ultrasound has proved to be of particular value in evaluating these cases. Conceptuses that are subsequently resorbed are frequently small in size for the gestational age and do not increase in diameter as rapidly as expected. It is not uncommon for small volumes of anechoic uterine luminal fluid to be identified before resorption. Smaller conceptuses are present in the uterine body for longer than normal because of their size. This may result in failure of maternal recognition of pregnancy. Other indicators of impending resorption are failure of fixation and orientation at the correct time. Following early embryonic loss, small volumes of fluid may be imaged within the uterine lumen; however, remnants of the conceptus are not identified.

From day 21 onwards, failure of embryonic development indicates impending pregnancy loss, although this should be interpreted with care in the case of multiple conceptuses where embryonic tissue is ofen imaged later than expected. The features of embryonic or fetal death are: an irregular outline of the conceptus and small size for the gestational age; increased echogenicity of the allantoic or yolk sac fluid; poor definition of the embryonic or fetal tissue; and the absence of a heart beat. Echogenic tissue with disorganized membranes may be imaged free floating within the conceptus and fluid may be identified within the uterine lumen. Subsequently, there is thickening and inward bulging of the uterine wall and loss of volume of the conceptus. Following breakdown of the conceptus, uterine fluid containing echogenic material may be identified and oedema of the uterine wall may also be noted (Fig. 3.10).

FETAL ABORTION

Abortion of fetuses associated with expulsion of material may occur from midpregnancy onwards. The initial ultrasound fin-

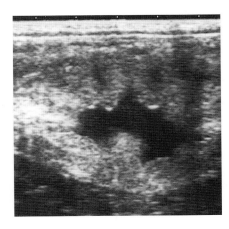

Fig. 3.10 Resorbing conceptus at day 20. There is collapse of the yolk sac and inward bulging of the uterine wall which appears oedematous. The previous day, the conceptus had appeared normal (7.5 MHz transducer, scale in cm).

dings are absence of the fetal heart beat, increased echogenicity of the fetal fluid and thickening of the uterine wall. The changes are similar to those identified with fetal resorption although it may be possible to identify caudal movement of fetal tissue and expulsion through the cervix. Following abortion, the uterus assumes an ultrasonographic appearance similar to that seen after parturition.

SUMMARY

An understanding of early embryological development and of the normal anatomy of the mare's reproductive tract allows the application of diagnostic ultrasound within clinical practice. Examination of the mare's reproductive tract with ultrasound facilitates the early diagnosis of pregnancy, the assessment of normal embryonic and fetal development, the confirmation of pregnancy viability and the diagnosis and management of pregnancy abnormalities, including multiple conceptuses.

FURTHER READING

Curran, S. S. (1992) Diagnosis of fetal gender by ultrasonography. In *Current Therapy in Equine Medicine*, 3rd edn. pp. 660–664. W. B. Saunders, Philadelphia.

Ginther, O. J. (1986) *Ultrasonic Imaging and Reproductive Events in the Mare.* Equiservices, Cross Plains, USA.

McKinnon, A. O., Voss, J. L., Squires, E. L. & Carnevale, E. M. (1993) Diagnostic ultrasonography. In *Equine Reproduction*, pp. 266–302. Lea & Febiger, Philadelphia.

Webbon, P. (1992) Ultrasound terminology. *Equine Veterinary Education* **4**, 286.

CHAPTER 4

Assessment and Management of Acute Trauma

CHARLES THURSBY-PELHAM

The word "trauma" is a transliteration from Greek and means a wound or bodily injury in general. The most common types of acute trauma which the general practitioner is likely to face are:

(1) Road traffic accidents.
(2) Falls.
(3) Lacerations and deeper wounds.
(4) Blows, e.g. from kicks.
(5) Burns.

The practitioner will usually be called to an emergency away from the clinic and so must take sufficient first aid equipment and be prepared to deal with a distraught client. The first aid equipment which should be readily to hand in the event of a call – to a road accident involving a horse, for example – is listed in Table 4.1. It may be necessary to have the materials for a Robert Jones bandage kept at the surgery and brought out to the horse if required (i.e. not all the kit will be carried in the car).

Table 4.1 First aid kit.

Sterile suture kit

10 rolls of cotton wool or gamgee

20 gauze bandages

Adhesive tape

2 half and 2 full limb splints (wooden boards, broom handles or light-weight metal), plastic gutter and saw

2 rolls of adhesive plaster, e.g. Elastoplast

Endotracheal/stomach tube and tracheotomy tube

14 G 9 cm catheters, giving set, three-way tap, heparin

Fluids:
  colloid, crystalloid, hypertonic (7.5%) saline

Needles:
  18 G 4 cm, 21 G 4 cm and 23 G 1.5 cm
Syringes:
  2.5, 10, 20 and 35 ml

Drugs:
  Adrenaline 1:1000
  NSAID, e.g. phenylbutazone, flunixin meglumine
  Corticosteroid (dexamethasone)
  Sedative, e.g. detomidine, xylazine, acepromazine
  Painkiller, e.g. butorphanol
  Anticonvulsant, e.g. diazepam
  Antibiotic, e.g. crystalline penicillin
  Tetanus antitoxin
  Local anaesthetic solution

Sterile dressings:
  petrolatum-impregnated gauze
  semiocclusive dressings

Gun and bullets

Headcollar and ropes

NSAID, non-steroidal anti-inflammatory drug.

INITIAL PROCEDURES

ON RECEIVING AN EMERGENCY CALL

Obtain a description of the location and nature of the emergency.

Obtain the name of the caller. If a police officer is present obtain his or her personal number and the station location.

Contact an equine practice and request assistance if you are unsure of being able to provide more than first aid.

ON ARRIVAL

Restrain the horse with a headcollar or bridle, even if the horse is recumbent or trapped.

Take charge. The owner is frequently more upset than the horse, and there is often a superfluity of bystanders all offering different advice. Keep all bystanders, except those of use to you, at a distance.

If possible, move the horse out of the way of traffic.

EMERGENCY EUTHANASIA

There are a number of alternatives available for euthanasia of the horse (see Chapter 1). The humane killer employing a free bullet is the most frequently used and is quick and practical. The recommended site is said to lie just above the intersection of two imaginary lines joining the base of the ears to the centre of the opposite orbits. In practice, it is easy to make the mistake of aiming too low than too high, and placing the muzzle of the gun just below the base of the forelock is quicker (and looks better to bystanders) than taking measurements. It is important to ensure that everyone is standing behind you, because the bullet can ricochet out of the side of the horse.

Of the intravenous agents, the mixture of quinalbarbitone and cinchocaine (Somulose, Arnolds) appears to be the most satisfactory, owing to the comparatively small volume required (see Chapter 1). It is, however, subject to the Misuse of Drugs Regulations 1985. Cutting the aorta per rectum is a last resort and is not recommended.

HISTORY

The initial history should be brief but give an indication of the systems that are likely to be involved. The time of the accident should be ascertained in order that the degree of shock and ability of the body to cope can be gauged.

INITIAL CLINICAL EXAMINATION

On arrival, a quick examination should be performed in order to identify and treat any life-threatening problems, e.g. severe respiratory or cardiovascular embarrassment. An "ABC of emergency" is described in Table 4.2 and drug dosages are listed in Table 4.3.

Table 4.2 ABC of emergency.

A   Airway

Ensure patency of the airway. Any obstructing fluids or objects should be removed from the airway and the horse intubated if necessary. If pulmonary oedema is evident, 10 ml of 50% ethanol can be given intratracheally. Intravenous clenbuterol is useful when fluid (whether inhaled or produced by the horse) is obstructing the lower respiratory tract. Emergency tracheotomy may be required to bypass an upper respiratory tract obstruction.

B   Breathing

Once the airway is patent, it may be necessary to artificially ventilate the horse by pressing on the thorax every 15 seconds. Oxygen is used if available. Doxapram hydrochloride (Dopram V, Willows Francis) may be beneficial.

C   Circulation

Stem any profuse haemorrhage by direct digital pressure, ligation, tourniquet, packing or bandaging. In the event of asystole, external cardiac massage should be performed at a rate of 40/minute. Following reoxygenation of the heart, adrenaline (0.5–1.0 ml of 1:1000 in 10 ml water for an adult horse) may be injected intravenously or into the heart. Intravenous fluids, if available, are given to expand the circulatory volume. Polyionic fluids are normally used but, if there has been excessive haemorrhage, then plasma volume expanders (e.g. Haemaccel, Hoechst) or whole blood (15–25 ml/kg) are appropriate. Blood may safely be transfused from a random donor without cross-matching on the first occasion and up to 8 litres may be safely removed from a healthy 500 kg horse. Recently, hypertonic saline (7.5%) has been advocated for the emergency treatment of horses in severe shock and is probably effective more quickly than colloids; 2–3 litres should be administered to a 500 kg horse, but this *must* be followed by the usual large volumes (20–40 litres) of isotonic solution within 1–2 hours.

Table 4.3 Emergency drug dosages.

Drug	Dose	Per 500 kg horse
Acepromazine	0.05–0.1 mg/kg IV or IM	2.5–5 ml of 10 mg/ml
Adrenaline 1:1000	0.2 ml/50 kg IM	2.4 ml IM 1 ml in 10 ml water IV or IC
Butorphanol	0.1 mg/kg IV	5 ml of 10 mg/ml 1 ml per 0.5 ml detomidine
Clenbuterol hydrochloride	1.25 ml/50 kg of 0.03 mg/ml	12.5 ml of 0.03 mg/ml
Detomidine	0.01–0.02 mg/kg IV or IM	0.5–1 ml of 10 mg/ml
Dexamethasone	5–20 mg IV or IM	10 ml of 2 mg/ml
Diazepam	5–10 mg (foals) IV 25–100 mg (horses) IV	100 mg
Flunixin meglumine	1.1 mg/kg IV or IM	10 ml of 50 mg/ml
Phenylbutazone	4.4 mg/kg IV	10 ml of 200 mg/ml
Romifidine 10 mg/ml	0.4–1.2 ml/100 kg IV	3–5 ml 2.5 ml and 1 ml butorphanol
Sodium benzylpenicillin	2.5–10 megaunits IV or IM	10 megaunits in 20 ml water
Tetanus antitoxin	3000 units prophylactically	
Trimethoprim 40 mg/ml ⎱ Sulphadiazine 200 mg/ml ⎰	1 ml/16 kg IM, or IV if aqueous solution	35 ml (not after detomidine)
Xylazine 20 mg/ml	3–5 ml/100 kg IV slowly	

IC, intracardially; IM, intramuscularly; IV, intravenously.

During the initial examination, note the state of consciousness, nature and quality of the pulse and respiration, mucous membrane colour, capillary refill time, temperature of the extremities and any gross musculoskeletal damage. Clinical improvement of hypovolaemia is demonstrated by a decreased

heart rate, increased pulse pressure, shorter capillary and jugular refill times, and warming of the extremities.

COMPREHENSIVE CLINICAL EXAMINATION

The horse will present with one or more of the following manifestations of acute trauma:

(1)   Recumbency.
(2)   Non-weightbearing lameness.
(3)   Severe dyspnoea.
(4)   Wounds.
(5)   Ocular emergencies.
(6)   Abdominal trauma.

RECUMBENCY

The recumbent horse is a diagnostic and therapeutic challenge.
A horse may be winded by a fall while galloping and jumping
and remain recumbent for half an hour before getting up and
being none the worse for wear. It is therefore vital that exhausted or winded horses are not euthanased prematurely. These
horses must be distinguished from those that are recumbent
and breathing hard as a result of head trauma or musculoskeletal damage to one or more limbs or the spine.

Differential diagnosis

(1)   Head trauma.
(2)   Spinal trauma.
(3)   Musculoskeletal damage to a limb or limbs.
(4)   Major blood vessel rupture.
(5)   Winded or exhausted.

Head trauma

There is usually direct or circumstantial evidence of head
trauma having occurred. A period of unconsciousness may

result and, where possible, euthanasia should not be performed for at least 24 hours, during which time appropriate diagnostic and therapeutic measures may be taken. Unconsciousness may be followed by depression, circling, seizures, facial desensitization, pupil asymmetry, depressed pupillary light reflexes, eye deviations and vestibular signs (Fig. 4.1). Ataxia and weakness may occur and the horse may relapse into recumbency again. In cases with severe or progressive neurological signs, bleeding from the nostrils or ears, and lacerations or fractures of the forehead, the practitioner should arrange for radiography of the skull to be performed.

Delirious or thrashing horses may be sedated with acepromazine. Xylazine and detomidine should be used with caution as they may increase the blood pressure (increasing central nervous system haemorrhage) and cause respiratory depression. Seizures are controlled with diazepam or, if severe, by general anaesthesia. Glucocorticoids are usually given if neurological signs follow cranial trauma (0.1–0.2 mg/kg dexamethasone every 4–6 hours for 1–3 days), but the horse should be monitored carefully for steroid-induced laminitis. A dose of 0.25–1 g/kg of 20% mannitol may be administered intravenously to unconscious horses and repeated after 6–12 hours if there is improvement. Flunixin meglumine or phenylbutazone will alleviate pain and oedema and improve demeanour but, with

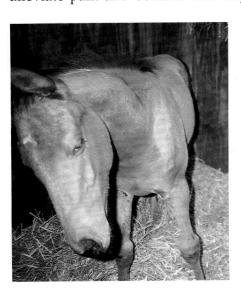

Fig. 4.1 A 6-month-old foal exhibiting head tilt following a 15-minute period of unconsciousness after going over backwards. The foal was blind, and euthanased 2 weeks later when optic nerve atrophy became apparent.

prolonged therapy, the horse should be monitored for signs of gastric ulceration and renal toxicity. It has been suggested that dimethyl sulphoxide (DMSO) may reduce central nervous system swelling and inflammation (1 g/kg of 10% DMSO in 0.9% saline intravenously, repeated up to six times in 3 days) but this is unproven (Pringle, 1992).

Spinal trauma

Spinal trauma can present as recumbency and may occur in association with head trauma or musculoskeletal injury. There is often localized or diffuse sweating and horses frequently struggle because of pain or their inability to stand. First aid comprises sedation of a thrashing animal with xylazine or diazepam and intravenous dexamethasone and phenylbutazone. A thorough neurological examination should be performed and, although the prognosis is guarded for a horse which is recumbent owing to spinal trauma, premature euthanasia should be avoided. Provided the horse is not in uncontrollable pain and does not have to be moved from the scene of the accident (frequently a priority that overrides all others at equestrian events) then a more accurate prognosis can be given after assessing the response to treatment over the next few hours. Time is a great healer of spinal injury and, providing there is no further damage, there may be a great improvement in neurological function (Mayhew, 1989). The horse should be kept warm with rugs and its legs bandaged.

The veterinarian, however, is frequently put under considerable pressure by course authorities and the public to make a rapid decision on euthanasia. Under these circumstances, he or she should still endeavour to make as full an examination as possible. Poor prognostic indicators include areflexia, extensor rigidity, shallow and rapid respiration that does not slow and deepen, the horse attaining a "dog-sitting" position, and a marked cut-off in sweating.

Limb damage

Musculoskeletal damage to the limbs, e.g. a fractured femur, may also present as recumbency. A lower limb injury is more likely to present as a non-weightbearing lameness but may be seen in a recumbent horse. For this reason, one should avoid moving a recumbent patient excessively until the possibility of an unstable fracture has been ruled out. If the horse is to be transported, it should be drawn into a trailer on a mat and positioned so that its head and neck can be supported with cushions; one should avoid pulling the legs, head or tail in so doing as this may cause further pain and aggravate a lesion (Deboer, 1992). The humanitarian grounds for such action – particularly in the eyes of the public – must be considered first.

NON-WEIGHTBEARING LAMENESS

Differential diagnosis

(1)   Fracture.
(2)   Tendon inflammation, rupture or laceration.
(3)   Luxation or subluxation.
(4)   Nerve damage, e.g. radial paralysis.
(5)   Septic joint or tendon sheath.
(6)   Foreign body or pus in the foot.

Fractures

First aid for fractures is aimed at providing adequate support to prevent the fracture compounding or further soft tissue damage. In order that a horse may be removed from a course, temporary support can be provided by applying a gutter splint (two lengths of foam-padded plastic guttering, 12–15 cm in diameter, taped around the leg). Once the horse is off the course a Robert Jones bandage or a rapid-setting resin cast is applied; the joints proximal and distal to the fracture should be immobilized, and a reinforced Robert Jones bandage is frequently used for the purpose (Fig. 4.2).

Pain is a protective mechanism and so, although it should be reduced on humane grounds, it should not be abolished completely. The pressure and immobilization provided by the Robert Jones bandage will reduce the pain and this can be supplemented with non-steroidal anti-inflammatory drugs (NSAIDs) and butorphanol. Sedation should be avoided as it

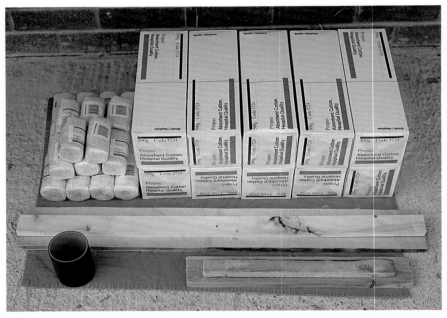

Fig. 4.2 Materials for a Robert Jones bandage. A Robert Jones bandage may cover the whole limb, in which case ten 500 g rolls of cotton wool and up to twenty gauze or crepe bandages may be used, or half the limb. One inch (2.5 cm) thick layers of cotton wool are applied and each layer is held firmly in place by gauze or crepe. Each layer is wrapped more tightly than the last until the total diameter is three times that of the leg. The bandage may be made more rigid by incorporating two splints at right angles to each other along its length; splints may comprise wood, PVC or lightweight metal, and are strapped over the bandage with adhesive tape. In cases of proximal radial and tibial fractures, the splint should extend proximally, on the lateral side of the limb, to the chest or upper thigh to prevent abduction (Schramme, 1989).

may result in incoordination and further injury, especially during transport.

A fracture patient should ideally be transported in a low-loading trailer or box, with the horse's head free and supported by bales. The injured limb should be positioned to the rear of the vehicle so that the sound limbs can absorb the relatively greater forces produced by braking as opposed to accelerating.

At the clinic, a full clinical and radiological assessment can be made before deciding on treatment and prognosis. As a general rule, long bone shaft fractures proximal to the carpus or tarsus in adult horses are almost certainly an indication for euthanasia. One aid to reaching such a diagnosis is that these fractures are often associated with the rapid formation of large intramuscular haematomata. Olecranon fractures are an exception and do not warrant emergency euthanasia (Fig. 4.3). There are reports of successful treatment of radial (Auer and Watkins, 1987) and tibial (Bramlage and Hanes, 1982) shaft fractures, but this is expensive and demands a high degree of expertise. If in doubt, a second opinion should be sought.

Tendon damage

Severe tendonitis, tendon rupture (the ends of superficial digital flexor tendon can often be palpated immediately following rupture) and laceration of the flexor tendons are most successfully treated by the application of a board cast (Fig. 4.4). The cast allows the weight to be borne through a vertical strut of bone and minimizes tension on the flexor tendons. The underlying pressure bandage minimizes further damage to the tendons through exudate accumulating and dissecting between torn and healthy fibres. Commercial splints, for example the Monkey splint (Kruuse UK Ltd, Sherburn-in-Elmet, North Yorks), are

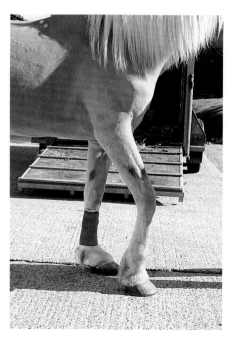

Fig. 4.3 Horse with olecranon fracture.

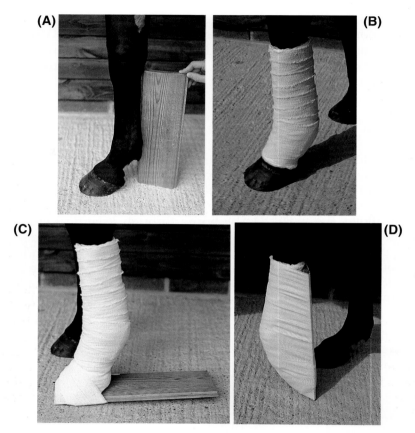

Fig. 4.4 Application of a board cast. (A) Cut a piece of wood to the width of the shoe and ground to knee height (measured against the unaffected leg). (B) Clean and dress any underlying wounds and apply a pressure bandage to the leg (a roll of gamgee or cotton wool and two elasticated bandages). (C) Strap one end of the board to the sole of the foot using a roll of elastic adhesive bandage. (D) Raise the other end of the board and strap it to the back of the leg, thereby placing the lower leg in forced flexion.

now available and are very effective. An NSAID and antibiotics (for open wounds) are also administered.

Luxations

Luxations may be complete or partial and involve disruption to one or more joint ligaments; there may also be an associated fracture. Lower limb luxations should be treated as fractures and evaluated at a clinic.

Nerve damage

Trauma to the lateral aspect of the humerus can result in radial nerve paralysis. Because the radial nerve supplies the extensors of the elbow, carpus and digit, the horse will stand with the elbow dropped and extended while the carpus and digit are flexed. The elbow muscles and the extensors of the digits will be relaxed and the limb will appear longer than normal. Although unable to advance the limb, the horse can bear weight if the foot is placed under it. The humerus, radius and ulna should be carefully examined for fractures in cases of radial paralysis. Occasionally, there may also be paralysis of the brachial plexus, resulting in flexor paralysis and a total inability to bear weight.

Femoral paralysis can follow a blow to the limb or may be caused by the horse slipping. The animal will be unable to bear weight and the joints of the affected limb will be flexed.

Trauma to the lateral aspect of the stifle can result in peroneal paralysis. Hyperextension of the hock and hyperflexion of the fetlock and digit cause the horse to drag the fetlock along the ground. Weight can be borne if the foot is placed under the horse, but the fetlock will knuckle as soon as walking is attempted.

There is no specific treatment for these injuries, except time: the minimum period before one might expect to see some improvement is 6 weeks.

Septic synovial structure

Sepsis in a synovial structure may result in a non-weightbearing lameness but this is usually insidious in onset. One should be careful that acute trauma does not progress to this. Treatment comprises repeated drainage and lavage of the structure and prolonged antibiotic therapy. Chronic cases may require surgical debridement and subtotal synovectomy.

Pus in the foot

The most common cause of sudden onset, severe lameness is subsolar abscessation. The horse will usually be found unwilling to bear weight on the affected limb. Pus in the foot can also manifest itself as severe lameness when a horse pulls up after a gallop. Infection gains entry to the foot via a puncture wound or a crack in the white line. The sole and white line should, therefore, be examined for black spots which should be probed to their depths. Applying pressure with hoof testers (under regional analgesia if necessary) can force the pus out of a hole. Occasionally, the condition is not noticed until the abscess ruptures out at the coronary band. Pus in the foot must be differentiated from a pedal bone fracture in which the pain is usually more severe and widespread over the sole. If in doubt, radiography should be arranged.

Treatment of pus in the foot involves drainage of the abscess followed by tubbing or poulticing (for 2 days) and then preventing contamination of the hole. Antibiotics are not indicated in uncomplicated cases but antitetanus cover should be ensured.

The consequences of penetration of the sole by a foreign body depend on the site, the depth and the direction of the penetration (Fig. 4.5). Penetrations of the middle-third of the sole are potentially the most serious as they may involve the navicular bone or bursa, the deep digital flexor tendon or the coffin joint. If a radiodense foreign body is still in place then, ideally, radi-

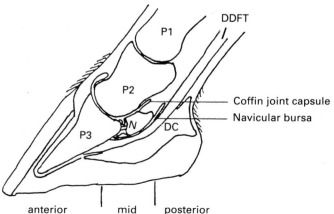

Fig. 4.5 Midsagittal section of the foot highlighting the danger areas for foreign body penetration. P1, first phalanx; P2, second phalanx; P3, third phalanx; N, navicular bone; DC, digital cushion; DDFT, deep digital flexor tendon.

ography should be performed with it in situ. Usually this is not practical, however, in which case the depth and angle of penetration should be gauged when the foreign body is removed. Subsequent radiography with and without a probe or contrast medium may be necessary. Arthrocentesis may be required to confirm involvement of the coffin joint.

Treatment depends on the above factors but would include tetanus prophylaxis, antibiotics, drainage and repeated flushing of the tract. Other therapy might consist of curettage of the pedal bone, drainage of the navicular bursa and lavage of the coffin joint. Where deeper structures are involved, owners should be warned that treatment can be prolonged and that the prognosis is guarded to poor.

SEVERE DYSPNOEA

Differential diagnosis

(1) Upper respiratory tract trauma:
     foreign body
     nasal trauma
     pharyngeal trauma
     mandibular trauma
     heat/smoke damage (stable fire)
(2) Lower respiratory tract trauma:
     fractured ribs
     penetrating wounds
     ruptured diaphragm (possible herniation of bowel into the thorax)
(3) Non-traumatic causes:
     chronic obstructive pulmonary disease
     strangles abscessation
     severe pain or shock
     guttural pouch tympany or empyema

Upper respiratory tract trauma

Severe dyspnoea arising from trauma is uncommon. Upper respiratory tract obstruction causes inspiratory dyspnoea and a patent airway must be established by nasotracheal intubation or, if necessary, by an emergency tracheotomy (Table 4.4). More commonly, foreign bodies in the oropharynx result in dysphagia, coughing and sometimes haemoptysis. The horse will tend to hold its head and neck extended, and the diagnosis can be confirmed by endoscopy. General anaesthesia is usually required for foreign body removal, which may be conducted either via the mouth or surgically (Greet, 1985).

Although trauma to the nasal cavity (e.g. nasal bone fracture) can result in dyspnoea, bleeding from the nose, an altered facial contour and subcutaneous emphysema are more typical presenting signs. Dyspnoea may occur up to a week after a stable fire (see below).

EMERGENCY TRACHEOTOMY

(1)   Infuse local anaesthetic solution subcutaneously in a 10 cm line along the ventral midline of the middle third of the neck.
(2)   Tensing the skin rostrally, incise through the skin and subcutaneous tissues along this line (Fig. 4.6).

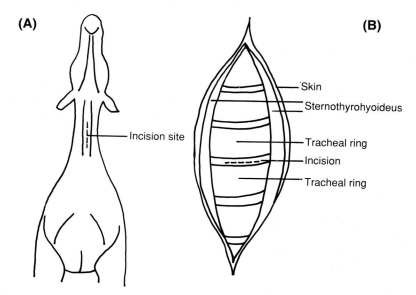

Fig. 4.6 Emergency tracheotomy. (A) Skin incision. (B) Site of insertion of tracheotomy tube.

(3) Bluntly divide the paired muscle bellies of sternothy-rohyoideus in the midline.
(4) Incise midway *between* two of the tracheal rings and extend the incision 1 cm either side of the midline. Insert the tracheo-tomy tube (Fig. 4.7).

Lower respiratory tract trauma

Alternatively, the lower respiratory tract may be traumatized. A direct blow is usually responsible for rib fractures and the horse presents with shallow, rapid breathing, pain and occasionally crepitus and subcutaneous emphysema over the affected ribs. Conservative treatment is usually sufficient. If pneumothorax develops (confirmed radiographically) suction drainage and fracture repair may be necessary. Penetrating wounds to the thorax may result in pneumothorax and pleurisy, such cases presenting with distressed breathing and symptoms of shock. General anaesthesia using intermittent positive press-ure ventilation and suction drainage are required for the repair of these wounds (Burbidge, 1982). Diaphragmatic rupture more commonly presents as abdominal distress (see below).

Non-traumatic causes

It is important to rule out more common causes of distressed breathing by thorough clinical examination; such causes include chronic obstructive pulmonary disease, strangles abscessation, pain and shock.

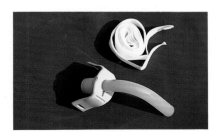

Fig. 4.7 Tracheotomy tube.

WOUNDS

Wounds may manifest as cuts, skin flaps, skin deficits, stake wounds, puncture wounds or burns. It is important to assess the depth and extent of the wound and which associated tendons, ligaments, bursae, joints or bones may be affected (Fig. 4.8). A minor skin wound may overlie a far more serious problem and so the wound should not be sutured until the underlying tissues have been assessed.

Wound evaluation

(1)   Severe bleeding is stemmed by applying pressure, haemostats, ligation or a tourniquet. Sedation is frequently required and, in the case of distal limb wounds, is followed by regional perineural anaesthesia; elsewhere, direct infiltration of the wound is acceptable, after it has been cleansed.
(2)   With the wound protected by sterile moist swabs or K-Y Jelly, the surrounding area is clipped or shaved and aseptically prepared.
(3)   The swabs are removed or the K-Y Jelly is flushed out along with any adherent hairs. The wound is lavaged with 0.1–0.2% povidone-iodine (1–2 ml in 1 litre sterile saline) and debrided, before a final rinse with sterile saline. Adequate pressure may be obtained by forcing the fluid through a 19 G needle using a 50 ml syringe.

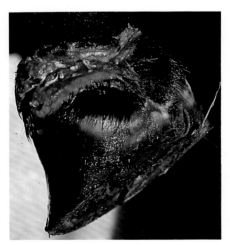

Fig. 4.8 A wire wound to the posterior pastern which penetrated the digital sheath.

(4)   Sterile gloves are worn to palpate the wound's depth, and a sterile instrument may be used to probe a tract in order to identify a foreign body or whether vital structures are affected. If so, radiography, possibly using contrast material, may be arranged.

(5)   Synovial fluid may be identified by stringing it between thumb and forefinger, or by cytology. If doubt exists as to whether a synovial structure has been penetrated then, after aseptic preparation, sterile saline may be introduced into the structure at a site remote from the wound, and the wound observed for the appearance of saline. If this occurs, then the needle is left in place and the structure lavaged with sterile saline. Synovial fluid quickly becomes grossly abnormal following contamination of a joint and a needle aspirate from a site removed from the wound will indicate whether immediate joint lavage is necessary.

Treatment

Once the wound has been evaluated, a decision as to whether to opt for wound closure (be it primary, delayed primary or secondary) or second intention healing must be made.

Primary closure is usually attempted for recent wounds, if there is minimal contamination and a good blood supply to the skin edges.

Delayed primary closure may be used on wounds involving a synovial structure and on those severely contaminated, contused or swollen.

Secondary closure is occasionally employed for chronic wounds with a poor blood supply, once a sufficient blood supply exists to support healing.

Second intention healing is selected for wounds with excessive tissue loss, and for large wounds of the upper limbs, body and neck (Fig. 4.9).

As most wounds are contaminated to some degree, it is advisable, if the wound is to be sutured, to leave a dependent drainage hole or to insert a drain. Drains are particularly useful if the wounds are more than skin deep, but should be removed within 4 days to prevent a foreign body reaction occurring. Tetanus cover must always be established and, if in doubt, antitoxin administered. Penicillin is a good first-line antibiotic for most wounds, but if a synovial structure is involved, a broader-

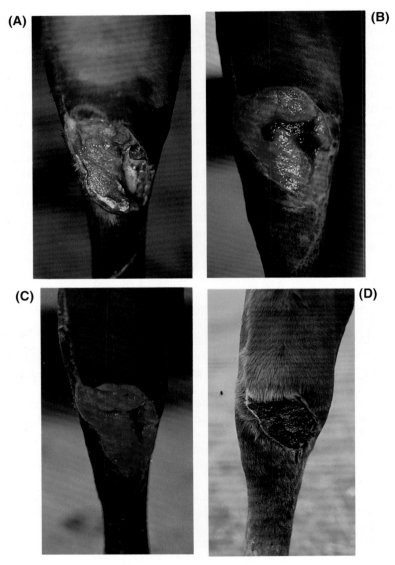

Fig. 4.9 Wound to the anterior aspect of the hock in a 2-year-old part-thoroughbred gelding. The proximal dorsal cannon was exposed and the periosteum torn. Radiography and arthrocentesis revealed no joint involvement or fracture. After debridement and lavage the wound was allowed to heal by second intention. Petrolatum gauze and absorbent bandage were used initially, followed by semiocclusive dressings under firm bandaging. Excision and corticosteroid ointment were used to control proud flesh.

spectrum antibiotic should be chosen, e.g. ampicillin or genta-micin in combination with penicillin. Potentiated sulphona-mides are useful for prolonged treatment (oral preparations are available).

Contaminated wounds of the limbs that are to heal by second intention should be bandaged. If copious discharge from the wound is anticipated, then petrolatum-impregnated gauze with an absorbent covering may be used initially, as this will draw the exudate away from the wound. Otherwise, a semiocclusive dressing which does not retard epithelialization, e.g. Melonin (Smith & Nephew), may be applied. Equine wounds, especially of the distal limb, are very prone to exuberant granulation tissue ("proud flesh").

There are considerable benefits to be gained from admitting severe wound cases to an equine clinic for surgical debridement and daily wound management.

Burns

When determining the severity and extent of burns sustained by a horse after a stable fire, say, the surface area of the burns should be measured. Two important points to bear in mind are:

(1) Full-thickness burns are four times more serious than partial-thickness ones (Table 4.4).
(2) Most horses die following severe burns to more than 50% of their body surface area and euthanasia should be considered in these cases.

The possible complications of severe burns include infection, hypotensive shock due to the loss of protein-rich fluid, intra-vascular haemolysis and haemorrhagic diathesis. Heat and

Table 4.4 Indicators of full-thickness and partial-thickness burns.

Full thickness	Partial thickness
Oedema	Oedema
Erythema	Analgesia
Hyperaesthesia	Avascularity
Exudation	Hair easy to pull out

smoke may damage the respiratory tract resulting in laryngitis, tracheitis, bronchopneumonia and pulmonary oedema, and such damage can take a week to manifest itself. Treatment includes broad-spectrum antibiosis, NSAIDs for pain relief, fluid replacement and wound management. Fluids low in potassium and high in sodium should be administered in sufficient quantities to ensure renal function without overhydrating (and so exacerbating pulmonary problems). Protein loss is initially combated with intravenous plasma or colloids and later by feeding alfalfa hay, methionine and moderate amounts of grain. Wounds should be clipped, cleansed with dilute antiseptic sterile saline and debrided before antiseptic or antibiotic ointment is applied (Stashak, 1991).

OCULAR EMERGENCIES

Where a horse has suffered trauma to the eyes or skull, a thorough examination of the eyes is essential, as the initial examination and treatment will affect the ultimate outcome of the injury. The horse will often be presented with blepharospasm, photophobia and lacrimation. In the first instance it is important not to touch the eyelids but to try to soothe the horse and see if it will open the eye(s) spontaneously (this time can be employed learning the history details). An attempt may then be made to open the lids. The orbicularis oculi muscles can make this very difficult; detomidine, given at sedative doses, is extremely useful in these circumstances and ophthalmological local anaesthetic drops may also be used. Tropicamide 1% (Mydriacyl, Alcon) is a short-acting mydriatic which allows more complete evaluation of the lens and posterior segment.

Eyelids

It is important to evaluate the globe when the eyelids are injured. Eyelid lacerations should be repaired promptly and accurate apposition of the eyelid margin is essential; minimal debridement should therefore be employed.

Globe

Traumatic proptosis is rare in the horse. If it occurs in association with severance of the optic nerve or severe damage to the globe then enucleation is indicated. If the extent of the damage cannot be determined the eye should be replaced and a temporary tarsorrhaphy performed; here, four to six interrupted horizontal mattress sutures are placed in the eyelids. Tension-relieving devices such as buttons may be used, but care should be taken not to penetrate the eyelid as the suture material would irritate the cornea.

Cornea

Superficial

Superficial corneal injuries may be treated medically. They should be stained with fluorescein to check for ulceration: uptake of the stain means that corticosteroids are contraindicated. The conjunctiva should be examined for the presence of a foreign body. Treatment comprises broad-spectrum topical antibiotic, 1% atropine drops and EDTA in water. The atropine

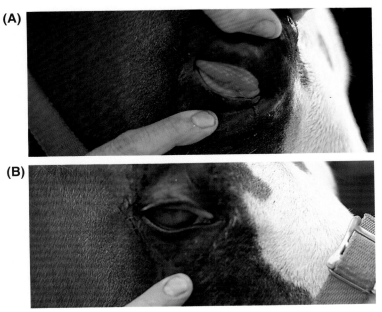

Fig. 4.10 Severe chemosis (A) in a pony which had had iodine splashed in its eye. The eye was lavaged with several litres of saline, EDTA drops were applied hourly and atropine every 4 hours; NSAIDs and antibiotics were administered. (B) Fluorescein staining revealed that the outer layers of the entire cornea had sloughed. Corneal epithelium could be seen migrating from the limbus after 2 days. A third eyelid flap with a subconjunctival chloromycin injection allowed re-epithelialization, and subsequent topical corticosteroids minimized neovascularization.

should be applied every 4 hours until the pupil dilates; although this will relieve any iritis, the owner should be warned that the pupil may not constrict in response to light for some weeks and the horse should be kept out of bright light until it does so. An EDTA blood tube filled with sterile water is a convenient, cheap and effective source of collagenase inhibitor and drops should be applied every 1–2 hours for the first day, if possible. Systemic and topical NSAIDs may also be used. Owners should be advised that direct sunlight, smoke, wind and flies will exacerbate keratitis. Chemical burns of the cornea should be copiously lavaged with water before instituting the above treatment (Fig. 4.10).

Deep

Deeper corneal lacerations may require suturing under general anaesthesia. Ointments should be avoided if corneal perforation is suspected because the petrolatum base can cause severe irido-cyclitis if it enters the anterior chamber (Brooks and Dan Wolf, 1984). Although superficial corneal foreign bodies can be removed under local anaesthesia and sedation, penetrating ones may require general anaesthesia and are probably best left to a veterinary ophthalmologist. Severe penetrating wounds should be referred as an emergency with topical and systemic antibiotic cover. If there is a delay then the eye may be protected in the meantime by a temporary tarsorrhaphy.

Uvea

Trauma to the eye often results in uveitis and so the eye should be examined in a dark area for signs of it. Treatment comprises topical atropine, corticosteroids, NSAIDs and antibiotics. Dexamethasone or NSAIDs may be given systemically.

ABDOMINAL TRAUMA

Fortunately, severe intra-abdominal trauma caused by external injury is uncommon in the horse. On the other hand, the consequences of contamination of the peritoneal cavity are even more serious than in other species.

Wounds

An abdominal wound should be explored (following aseptic preparation) by sterile digital palpation or sterile probing to identify its depth, any foreign body involvement and whether the peritoneal cavity has been penetrated. Rectal examination and abdominocentesis may be helpful if penetration is suspected.

Ultrasonography may be used to outline an embedded object. If a foreign body is suspected of having entered the peritoneal cavity, before it is removed, facilities should be available to deal with an ensuing visceral herniation. Wounds involving the peritoneal cavity are best managed under general anaesthesia with negative suction drainage and rigorous aseptic technique. Even with intensive antibiosis the prognosis would be guarded and with gross contamination euthanasia should be considered.

Wounds that do not penetrate the peritoneal cavity are managed in the usual way.

Blunt trauma

Differential diagnosis

(1) Rupture of abdominal viscus.
(2) Internal haemorrhage.
(3) Rupture of abdominal wall.
(4) Ruptured diaphragm.

Investigation

Historical evidence in conjunction with clinical signs of shock and possibly colic may suggest such problems. Rectal examination and abdominocentesis may help the diagnosis: contamination of the peritoneal cavity with gut contents gives the intestines a granular feel on rectal examination and peritoneal fluid would be green-brown and cloudy (as opposed to the normal clear yellow). Enterocentesis will also yield such fluid. Confirmation of a ruptured bowel is an indication for immediate euthanasia.

Fresh blood may be obtained by abdominocentesis in cases of internal haemorrhage. If, on the other hand, the first few drops are blood-tinged and then the fluid clears, a blood vessel may have been punctured. Splenic puncture may also occur. Internal haemorrhage may be treated conservatively with blood transfusion, colloids and crystalloids, or surgically.

In cases of traumatic rupture of the abdominal muscles, a loop of bowel may be felt passing into the hole. If the rupture is in the form of a gridiron tear, however, a hernial ring cannot be identified and so diagnosis and reduction of herniated bowel is difficult. Immediate surgery is indicated in cases of incarcerated bowel; in the absence of incarceration, surgery should be delayed until infection and inflammation are under control.

Clinical signs of diaphragmatic rupture include colic, which may manifest as recurrent bouts, tachypnoea, dyspnoea, borborygmi audible in the chest (difficult to interpret) and dullness of the caudoventral thorax on the affected side. Diagnosis is confirmed by thoracic radiography or laparotomy. There are reports of repair of diaphragmatic rupture (Scott and Fishback, 1976) but the surgery is difficult and should not be undertaken lightly.

Performing a peritoneal tap

(1) Clip and scrub a 10 cm wide strip from xiphisternum to umbilicus.
(2) Insert a 19 G 5 cm needle through the skin at the lowest point of the abdomen.
(3) Gently advance the needle through the linea alba.
(4) Collect the fluid in an EDTA tube.
(5) If no fluid appears twist the needle – it can take some time. If necessary, try cranial or caudal to this site. A longer needle or catheter may be required for fat horses.

GENERAL TIPS

ASSISTING A HORSE TO RISE

It is not possible to lift an adult horse to its feet by manpower alone: one can only assist the horse and optimize its efforts. A horse that has fallen on a slippery surface should be manoeuvred so that any slope in the ground can be used to its advantage: it should be faced downhill or, failing that, its hind-legs should be directed downhill. The front feet are pulled out forwards and placed on a non-slip surface, e.g. rubber car mats. One person pulling the tail upwards and one on the headcollar rope are usually all that are necessary, but a weak animal may benefit from two people either side supporting it with a broad sling. Someone standing on the dorsal hoof walls of the front feet as the horse attempts to rise also helps.

All human efforts should be reserved for when the horse makes its big effort. A certain amount of goading may be necessary to encourage this.

REMOVING A HORSE FROM A DITCH OR BOG

Assuming there is no musculoskeletal injury, the horse should be orientated so as to optimize its own efforts. If it has become wedged upside down in a ditch then it should be rolled into sternal recumbency so that it can get itself up and walk out of the ditch. This may be achieved by means of a rope under its withers, ropes attached to each front leg (padded) and a halter rope, all pulling the horse's front end over its back end.

A horse that is stuck in a bog should not be pulled out forwards because this will tend to drive the front legs in deeper; equally, it should not be pulled by its head as this will damage the neck. A rope (or, preferably, a sling) should be passed around the chest behind the withers and the horse pulled out spine first. This will pull the legs out of the mud. The horse may then be dragged across the mud (on which horses float surprisingly well) to terra firma.

TRAILER ACCIDENTS

Horses – in marked contrast to their owners – are often surprisingly calm when in a trailer or horsebox that has turned over. A sedative may be administered as required; if minimal doses are given then the horses will be less likely to stand on each other when they get up. Headcollars should be fitted before any obstructing partitions are removed, and attempts should be made to try to soothe the horse before encouraging it to its feet.

Acknowledgements

The author wishes to thank Ian Camm and Robin Thursby-Pelham for their advice.

REFERENCES AND FURTHER READING

Auer, J. A. & Watkins, J. P. (1987) The treatment of radial fractures in adult horses: an analysis of 15 cases. *Equine Veterinary Journal* **19**, 103–110.

Bramlage, L. R. & Hanes, G. E. (1982) Internal fixation of a tibial fracture in an adult horse. *Journal of the American Veterinary Medical Association* **180**, 1090–1094.

Brooks, D. E. & Dan Wolf, E. (1984) Ocular trauma in the horse. *Equine Veterinary Journal* (Supplement) **2**, 141–146.

Burbidge, H. M. (1982) Penetrating thoracic wound in a Hackney mare. *Equine Veterinary Journal* **14** (1), 94–95.

Deboer, S. (1992) Transporting horses with severe leg or body injuries. *Equine Veterinary Education* **4** (1), 47–49.

Dyson, S. (1996) *A Guide to the Management of Emergencies at Equine Competitions*. British Equine Veterinary Association, 5 Finlay Street, London SW6 6HE.

Greet, T. R. C. (1985) The respiratory tract. In *Equine Surgery and Medicine* (ed. J. Hickman), pp. 247–296. Academic Press, New York.

Mayhew, I. G. (1989) *Large Animal Neurology*. Lea & Febiger, Philadelphia.

Pringle, J. (1992) Emergency treatment of the traumatised horse. In *Current Therapy in Equine Medicine 3*, (ed. N. E. Robinson). W. B. Saunders, Philadelphia.

Schramme, M. C. (1989) The Robert Jones bandage. *Equine Veterinary Education* **1**, 50–51.

Scott, E. A. & Fishback, W. A. (1976) Surgical repair of diaphragmatic hernia in a horse. *Journal of the American Veterinary Medical Association* **168**, 45–47.

Stashak, T. S. (1987) *Adams' Lameness in Horses*. Lea & Febiger, Philadelphia.

Stashak, T. S. (1991) *Equine Wound Management*. Lea & Febiger, Philadelphia.

Wyn-Jones, G. (1988) *Equine Lameness*. Blackwell Scientific Publications, Oxford.

CHAPTER 5

Equine Colic – To Refer or Not to Refer?

MARK JOHNSTON

The differentiation between cases of equine colic that can be treated medically and those that require surgery is a dilemma that worries even experienced equine veterinary surgeons. This chapter surveys the methods currently available to assist the clinician in the field dealing with a horse showing abdominal pain (Fig. 5.1).

Moore (1986) noted that horses exhibiting the cardinal signs of pain unresponsive to analgesic therapy, discoloured peritoneal fluid with a high protein content and tightly distended intestines per rectum do not provide a diagnostic dilemma, but this combination of clinical signs seems to be the exception rather than the rule.

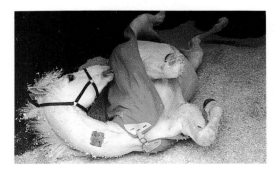

Fig. 5.1 The signs of abdominal pain pose a diagnostic dilemma for the veterinary surgeon.

If a diagnosis is not possible at the first visit, the examination should be repeated if possible at intervals of no more than 2 hours and the findings compared with those of the previous examinations. During this time it is important to avoid the use of flunixin meglumine as it may mask several of the signs on which recognition of the surgical case is based and lead to a fatal delay in embarking on surgery.

Although there have been many instances where adhesions, peritonitis and other postoperative complications have made the effects of surgery worse than the original disease, substantial advances in surgical and anaesthetic techniques have enabled many more patients with surgical lesions to be treated with a greater chance of success (Figs 5.2 and 5.3). However,

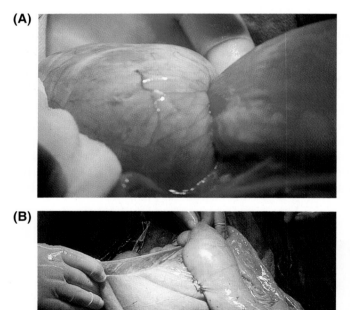

(A)

(B)

Fig. 5.2 Ileal-ileal intussusception (A), treated by side-to-side stapled anastomosis of ileum to caecum (B).

this progress has not been matched by advances in diagnostic procedures. The large size of equine patients has precluded the use of many of the newer and more exciting diagnostic methods adopted in human medicine. Hence the decision to operate remains difficult.

Misjudgements may occasionally occur when clinicians decide to operate to relieve a supposed surgical lesion and have negative surgical findings, but these will be less costly in terms of patient mortality than if surgery is delayed too long. By the time the clinician has appreciated the need for surgical intervention and persuaded the owner to transfer the horse to a clinic for colic surgery, it may indeed be too late (Fig. 5.4). The middle course between waiting too long and acting too quickly in sending a colic for surgery needs to be adopted. This path is difficult to chart and must rely on the individual referring veterinary surgeon's skill and experience. However, delay in deciding whether to refer an animal with abdominal pain or not can be the difference between life and death for the patient, so "if in doubt, send it". No surgical team will ever mind seeing a horse that was in severe pain but improved during transit and no longer demands surgical intervention.

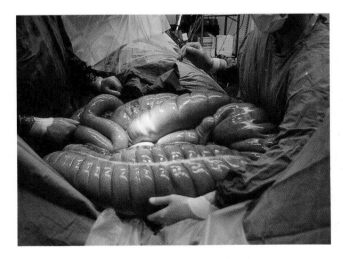

Fig. 5.3 Surgical correction of a colon torsion.

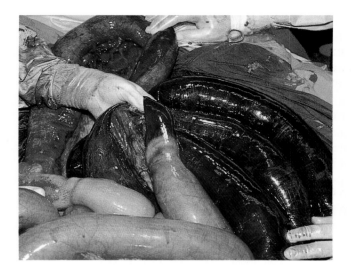

Fig. 5.4 Incarceration of small intestine through the epiploic foramen, referred too late for treatment.

DECISION IN THE FIELD

In deciding whether a case is surgical, there is no single criterion that can be relied on. All the information that circumstances permit should be gathered and weighed, so that a prognosis as well as a preliminary diagnosis can be suggested. The relevant points that should be considered when taking a history in these cases are listed below.

HISTORY

At grass

Very few non-surgical colics occur in animals permanently at grass. Grass sickness should appear on the list of differential diagnoses for any obstructive lesion in an animal at grass, as should infarctive disease resulting from intestinal parasitism.

Worming history

Many believe that a substantial number of colics remain worm-related. It thus makes sense to inquire about the anthelmintic regimen employed.

Age of the animal

Animals are susceptible to certain disorders according to their age: e.g. retained meconium in neonates, small intestinal caecal intussusceptions in foals and yearlings, colon torsions in recently foaled mares and pedunculated lipomas in older animals.

Breed or type

The larger breeds of horse are prone to large bowel displacements, such as nephrosplenic entrapment.

Stage of work

Often a horse that has suddenly come out of exercise and been confined to its box will experience low-grade abdominal pain. Most such cases are pelvic flexure impactions that require little more than medical therapy. Conversely, inguinal hernias in stallions are frequently associated with a history of recent exercise or covering a mare.

Previous episodes of colic

Repeated bouts of colic seldom occur without good reason. These reasons tend not to be medical and can be caused by a partial obstruction (e.g. tumour, abscess or enterolith) or by an intermittent obstruction such as an intussusception or a non-strangulating pedunculated lipoma. It is imperative that the animal is completely re-evaluated at each visit. It would not be the first time that a simple pelvic flexure impaction has subsequently developed into a colon torsion.

When was colic first noticed?

Animals found with abdominal pain first thing in the morning give cause for great concern, because the time of onset is uncertain. Irreversible changes in the gut wall can occur very quickly after vascular occlusion in both small and large intestine and it is rare for cases to be referred early enough for resection to be unnecessary. As soon as resection is carried out, the prognosis worsens considerably.

How rapidly has the patient deteriorated?

A rapid deterioration of clinical signs is consistent with irreversible intracellular changes, but precise information may not be available if the animal has only been under infrequent supervision.

CLINICAL EXAMINATION

Particular attention should be paid to the gastrointestinal and cardiovascular systems, as deterioration of cardiovascular function frequently accompanies intestinal ischaemia. Careful assessment of the vital signs, described below, together with the duration of the condition can give a relatively accurate appreciation of the underlying problem.

Pulse rate and quality

Edwards (1985) noted that pulse rate is more influenced by haemoconcentration, reduced venous return and endotoxaemia (all of which may be present) than by pain, which has a surprisingly minor effect on the pulse rate. Hence, intestinal infarction is usually accompanied by a non-fluctuating elevation in pulse rate, which tends to increase further as septic shock develops.

In some cases of colic, the circulation may be so compromised that the pulse is too weak to be appreciated and use of a stethoscope is indicated to measure heart rate. Conversely, the patient may be in such pain that it will not stand still long enough for its pulse or heart rate to be taken accurately.

Pulse strength is a subtle but important sign to assess, if the animal is not too violent, and gives a rough guide to peripheral blood pressure. A weak and easily compressible pulse is an indication of significant circulatory weakness. The pulse rate during a painful spasm is elevated by sympathetic nervous discharge and will quickly return to normal once the spasm relaxes. It is the pulse rate between spasms, and with adequate analgesia, that indicates the degree of circulatory compromise (i.e. areas of ischaemic gut) and the immediate need for surgery.

Mucous membrane colour

Reddening mucous membranes indicate developing haemoconcentration which is especially obvious in the terminal stages of endotoxic shock, because of vasodilatation of the capillary beds. Brick-red membranes are indicative of a need for surgery, if other criteria are met. A cyanotic tinge to already reddened membranes suggests a very poor prognosis.

Capillary refill time

Capillary refill time (CRT) is best assessed from the oral mucous membranes by applying brief digital pressure and noting the time taken to regain the previous colour. This should be done in conjunction with assessing the temperature of the extremities (ears and limbs). These two parameters taken together are supposedly accurate indicators of the state of the peripheral perfusion.

A CRT greater than 3 seconds, with cool extremities, is deemed abnormal and suggestive of inadequate peripheral perfusion and excessive vascular tone or vasoconstriction. However, peripheral capillaries are perfused by the hydrostatic pressure of fluid within the circulation just as much as by the direct support of the cardiovascular system, and the author has noticed, with some alarm, that dead horses can have almost normal capillary refill times.

Respiration

Rapid and shallow respirations may indicate an acute problem with developing toxaemia and metabolic acidosis (Edwards, 1985).

Abdominal distension

Abdominal distension is of little value in differentiating between medical and surgical colics, but is more indicative of the site of the lesion. It is only when there is gross distension of bowel distal to the ileocaecal valve that there is noticeable abdominal enlargement in the adult horse. This is especially obvious in the case of 360° colon torsion when the whole abdomen appears to blow up rapidly like a balloon. If there is little or no enlargement, then the obstruction is more likely to be oral to the ileocaecal valve.

Body temperature

A grossly elevated temperature can suggest a non-surgical problem, e.g. colitis or peritonitis.

Degree of pain

Pain, experienced before applying analgesia, can be subdivided into two types – visceral and parietal (Edwards, 1985). Its assessment is very subjective and owners have varying degrees of appreciation as to how much pain the animal has been experiencing. Quiet and careful questioning of the owner or handler is vital to extract the actual behaviour of the animal (scraping, rolling, throwing itself on the floor) rather than emotional descriptions of "agony". Individuals animals, furthermore, have different pain thresholds – a pony may show mild abdominal discomfort with a surgical lesion that would have a thoroughbred rolling around in agony.

(1) *Visceral pain* is mediated via the sympathetic nervous system and usually results from increased peristalsis, spasm, ischaemia and tension on the mesentery. Affected animals exhibit the classical signs of restlessness, kicking at the abdomen, scraping, lying down and rolling. External abdominal pressure is not usually resented unless over the affected viscus.
(2) *Parietal pain* is mediated via the somatic nervous system and is shown in any condition where there is inflammation of the parietal peritoneum, e.g. caused by intestinal contents leak-

ing from a perforation or rupture of a viscus. With this type of pain the patient tends to become immobile and external abdominal pressure is greatly resented wherever it is applied. The acuteness and severity of the pain depends on the degree of contamination of the abdominal cavity and the nature of the intraluminal contents (i.e., stomach rupture, releasing acidic contents, is much worse than rupture of the small colon or rectum) (Stashak, 1982).

Whether there is a single bout of agony or severe, unrelenting visceral pain, it is an important diagnostic sign, taken in conjunction with the physiological signs (cardiovascular status and degree of hydration). A rapid deterioration of physiological parameters and constant pain are strongly indicative of significant impairment of intestinal blood supply. Worsening of cardiovascular status, with a slight decrease in the amount of pain, can lull the owner and referring veterinary surgeon into believing that the horse is recovering, when in reality the intestines have just started to undergo gangrenous changes or have ruptured (Edwards, 1985).

Unremitting pain in the face of potent analgesics, such as pethidine, methadone, butorphanol or flunixin meglumine, strongly indicates the need for surgical intervention.

Gut sounds

Normal or increased borborygmi are inconsistent with major tissue changes and such cases tend to respond to medical therapy alone. It is the persistent absence of borborygmi that indicates a possible surgical lesion (this may develop subsequent to episodes of hypermotile gut sounds with an intussusception which has subsequently become strangulated). However, reduced borborygmi are a feature of a few medical conditions such as grass sickness or hypocalcaemia/hypokalaemia, or a passive gut obstruction, such as pelvic flexure impaction. Furthermore, such cases with no borborygmi are often those found to suffer from paralytic ileus if (or when) they come to surgery (Edwards, 1985).

It should be noted that the younger animal with distended small intestines and exhibiting hyperactive gut sounds (proximal to the suspected lesion) can indicate the presence of an intussusception, which may need bypass surgery.

Stomach tube placement and gas or fluid reflux

The technique of gastric reflux via stomach tube, well described by Urquhart (1987), has diagnostic and therapeutic value and should always be performed as part of the examination of any horse with colic. The relatively small size, unique orientation and strength of the cardia of the horse's stomach mean it is extremely unlikely that gas or fluid will exit via the oesophagus before the stomach ruptures (Moore, 1986). Adequate measures, and time, should be employed to ensure that gastric reflux caused by excessive intragastric pressure is removed. This can be achieved by lowering the patient's head and priming the indwelling stomach tube with water, developing a siphon by placing and maintaining the proximal end of the tube under water, altering the position of the stomach tube and persisting for 5–10 minutes before sequestrated fluid is obtained. The equine stomach has unpredictable qualities. It is not uncommon for a patient suffering from an upper small intestinal obstruction to have a stomach overfilled with fluid; yet when an indwelling stomach tube is positioned and charged with water to enable siphonation of the gastric contents, no reflux is obtained.

Medication by stomach tube should be avoided unless a specific diagnosis has been made (e.g. liquid paraffin for a pelvic flexure impaction) and no reflux has been obtained (Hunt, 1987).

Gastric reflux via stomach tube, of the retrieval of medication administered several hours earlier, indicates delayed gastric emptying or impaired or totally inhibited aboral fluid passage from stomach and small intestine. A primary small intestinal surgical obstruction or ileus (e.g. grass sickness, anterior enteritis) will be indicated by at least 2 litres of gastric reflux (Edwards, 1991). Dyspnoea and spontaneous regurgitation reflect severe gastric dilatation (Edwards, 1985).

Although the presence of an indwelling stomach tube in the stomach is said to reduce peristalsis and lead to ileus, this is more than outweighed by the benefit of having the stomach and small intestine at least partially decompressed when the patient comes to surgery.

Rectal examination

Examination per rectum is well described by Hunt (1987) and is the single most important aspect of the clinical examination of the horse with abdominal pain (Moore, 1986). However, its findings should not be considered in isolation from the rest of the clinical examination. The history and clinical signs may give the examiner guidance as to where abnormal rectal findings may be located and correctly differentiate between medical and surgical colic cases. It may be necessary to perform rectal examinations at intervals of 1–2 hours, especially at the start of the episode of colic. The examination should attend to each accessible area and be carried out in a thorough and systematic way. The normal landmarks should be appreciated (caudal pole of left kidney, caudal edge of spleen lying next to left body wall, pelvic flexure lying in the midline ventrally, the lack of palpable small intestine, normal position and size of caecum on the right side, ovaries, patent inguinal rings and bladder) and any abnormal structures described, to enable changes in such suspected lesions to be detected in later examinations.

Normal intestinal contractions may result in taut taenial bands of the large intestine. However, prolonged tautness of these bands over several hours combined with continued pain may indicate a large bowel displacement (Hunt, 1987). It is essential to avoid iatrogenic rupture of the rectum since this will severely prejudice the animal's chance of survival irrespective of the original cause of the colic.

Often only the caudal 30% of the abdomen can be reached in the most co-operative of adult horses and so this direct assessment of the state of the intestines can be less comprehensive than one would like. Small ponies and foals are often too small to allow rectal examination and it can be difficult and unsafe to examine patients in severe pain in this manner. However, sedation with 100–200 mg xylazine intravenously enables most patients to be examined per rectum. This sedative, aside from its analgesic benefit against abdominal pain (which often lasts longer than its sedative effect), is short-lived and unlikely to interfere with any potential premedication should the need for surgery arise.

Some specific findings that are indicative of the need for surgery are:

(1) Tightly distended loops of small intestine.
(2) Grossly distended large colon.
(3) Distended loop of small intestine leading to an inguinal ring.
(4) Nephrosplenic entrapment of the large colon.
(5) Palpable mass such as an enterolith.

The length of the small intestinal mesentery allows the small bowel to occupy any part of the abdomen from the pelvis to the diaphragm (Edwards, 1991) and small intestinal lesions are less easily definable, as proximal and distal small bowel feel the same per rectum. A loop of distended small intestine curling over the dorsal aspect of the caecum can be suggestive of duodenal involvement but this is often obscured by other loops of small intestine. Traction on the medial band of the caecum can sometimes elicit pain when the distal ileum is caught in a strangulating site such as the epiploic foramen. Distended small intestine is precise as a diagnosis in itself, indicating surgical interference, unless pyrexia ($> 40\,°C$) is present; this may be more indicative of an enteritis, e.g. salmonellosis (Hunt, 1987).

The catastrophe of an intestinal rupture reveals itself by a roughened and gritty sensation instead of the usually silky smooth feel of the serosal surfaces of the various structures of the abdomen. Once felt, it is never forgotten, and euthanasia should be carried out without delay.

Paracentesis abdominis

Paracentesis abdominis is performed as follows:

(1) A small midline area is clipped and scrubbed just caudal to the sternum.
(2) A 19 G 5 cm needle is inserted through the body wall at 90° to the skin and gently introduced into the peritoneal cavity. Fluid should flow from the needle hub and can be collected in EDTA or plain tubes for haematological and biochemical analysis.
(3) If no fluid is obtained, the needle can be lightly twisted by the fingertips to encourage flow. If there is still no fluid, further attempts can be made more caudally along the midline.

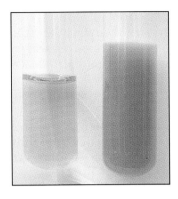

Fig. 5.5 Normal yellow peritoneal fluid (left). Abnormal homogeneous red peritoneal fluid (right), reflecting intestinal ischaemia.

(4)   Overweight patients can have excessive fat deposits under the linea alba which prevent sampling of the peritoneal fluid. In such cases, catheters up to 10 cm long are sometimes required to reach the peritoneal fluid. Extra care should be taken when using catheters of such length, to avoid intestinal puncture. Ultrasound has been helpful in assessing the depth of abdominal fat and in locating peritoneal fluid pockets.

Peritoneal fluid reflects the condition of the serosal surfaces of the structures in the abdomen (unless a structure is isolated in a pocket) and assists in assessing the status of any diseased bowel.

Often a simple visual inspection of the fluid may be all that is required (Figs 5.5, 5.6). Normal peritoneal fluid is yellow and clear. Peritonitis causes an increase in leucocytes and the fluid

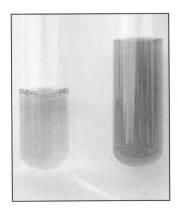

Fig. 5.6 Normal yellow peritoneal fluid (left). Green-brown discoloured fluid (right), reflecting intestinal rupture.

is more turbid and grey-white. Gut infarction is followed by both red and white cells entering the peritoneal cavity; the fluid is more sanguineous and turbid and the prognosis much worse. If the first few drops appear blood-tinged but this then clears, blood vessel puncture should be suspected and fluid collection from the needle hub reserved until the fluid colour is more consistent.

The presence of gut contents can indicate either perforated bowel or enterocentesis (Hunt, 1987). The presence of white blood cells in such a sample is likely to indicate a genuine gut rupture, with the ingesta mixing with peritoneal fluid.

Blood contamination of the sample is especially likely when the spleen is enlarged or displaced towards the midline, e.g. in nephrosplenic entrapment (Hunt, 1987).

Turner *et al.* (1984) reported that paracentesis fluid was the most helpful indicator of the need for surgery in 10 out of 15 cases of epiploic foramen incarceration. The usual reliable signs, such as pain, gastric reflux and palpable small intestinal distension per rectum, were not found in these cases which consistently revealed serosanguineous peritoneal fluid with an absolute white blood cell count greater than 10 000 cells/mm^3, and relative neutrophilia and total protein greater than 2.5 g/dl, indicating the presence of a strangulating intestinal lesion.

However, it is a mistake to place too much reliance on peritoneal fluid evaluation, since there have been many instances when non-viable gut has been found at surgery although the characteristics of the peritoneal fluid were normal (Moore, 1986). The author's experience supports these findings.

Laparotomy

A laparotomy subsequent to one or more attempts at obtaining a peritoneal fluid sample can demonstrate that paracentesis abdominis is not without risk. It is sobering to see the trauma that a 19 G needle can do to a distended section of small intestine and encourages one to be a little more cautious when penetrating the patient's abdomen, especially in foals and small ponies (Fig. 5.7).

Every effort should be made to refer horses with colic of unknown aetiology before the peritoneal fluid evaluation has changed. If one obtains serosanguineous fluid on the peritoneal

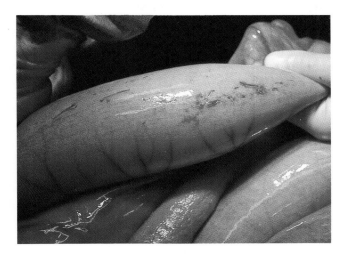

Fig. 5.7 Iatrogenic damage to small intestine by paracentesis abdominis using a 19 gauge needle.

tap, despite the possibility that it may be blood contaminated, one should be strongly suspicious that there is an intra-abdominal focus of intestinal ischaemia demanding surgical intervention (Edwards, 1991).

FIELD HAEMATOLOGY

Many colic cases progress to a degree of circulatory shock due to dehydration, hypovolaemia and endotoxaemia. This results in a relative polycythaemia. The consequent decrease in tissue perfusion can lead to metabolic acidosis, azotaemia and disruptions to the normal homeostasis of the blood clotting cascade. Packed cell volume (PCV) is probably the most frequently used laboratory test to suggest the ultimate prognosis and need for surgery. In general, a PCV above 60% caries a poor prognosis, whereas one below 35% carries a much better outlook.

However, the packed cell volume may be elevated by pain or excitement owing to splenic contraction. It is thus better to consider a raised PCV in conjunction with elevated total protein levels rather than a PCV value on its own, as a measure of intravascular dehydration and hence the need for fluid therapy. The use of battery-powered microcentrifuges enables a PCV value to be obtained in the field. Total protein assessment can also be achieved with refractometry.

RESPONSE TO ANALGESIA

A primary responsibility in the management of colic is the control of pain, but analgesic drugs should be chosen judiciously.

Xylazine/detomidine

Xylazine and detomidine are both sedatives which are known also to produce profound visceral analgesia (detomidine > xylazine, Thurmon 1990). A neuroleptanalgesic combination of xylazine/detomidine with butorphanol produces a synergistic benefit in visceral analgesia while allowing a reduced dose of xylazine.

The action of xylazine/detomidine is also to decrease gut motility by stimulating α_2-adrenergic receptors to increase transit time, although these are mild effects and of short duration. However, the concern by Clark and Becht (1987) that repeated doses of both of these drugs can reduce motility and either effectively downgrade the status of the patient, or delay the return of normal motility, is not supported by Rose and Rose (1988). The shorter duration of action of xylazine may interfere less with the subsequent induction of general anaesthesia and hence makes it the drug of choice in this situation.

Flunixin meglumine

Moore (1986) drew attention to the extra ability of flunixin meglumine, a cyclo-oxygenase inhibitor, compared with other NSAIDs (phenylbutazone, dipyrone and ibuprofen) to counteract the circulatory effects of endotoxins. The clinical responses (vasoconstriction, platelet aggregation, reduced tissue perfusion, pulmonary perfusion, pulmonary hypertension and abdominal pain) to a life-threatening ischaemic lesion of the bowel can be greatly reduced by administration of flunixin meglumine and lull the clinician into a false sense of security about the degree of state of the cardiovascular system.

Flunixin meglumine can be the referring veterinary surgeon's worst friend. It should only be used when a definite diagnosis is possible of a non-surgical colic or when the patient is committed to surgery and needs further analgesia. It is not as fast in onset as xylazine or butorphanol, but if flunixin meglumine has been given and the patient is still in pain a few minutes later, a decision should be made quickly either to transport it for immediate surgery or to consider euthanasia. However, a simple tympanitic episode may be so painful that it needs all analgesics available and benefits from flunixin meglumine.

Flunixin meglumine's Achilles heel has often first shown itself at this stage in the clinical examination. Colic cases that have been given flunixin meglumine may look deceptively good. The drug is particularly potent against the prostaglandin releasing effects of endotoxins in cases of strangulating intestinal lesions. The result is that the pulse rate and colour of mucous membranes may look satisfactory, but the peritoneal fluid is a homogeneous pink/red colour. The presence of a strangulating lesion of the intestines is very likely to be confirmed at surgery. Such experiences have restricted the author's use of flunixin meglumine to colics where a definite non-surgical diagnosis (e.g. pelvic flexure impaction) has been made, and to cases where all other analgesics have failed and the animal is being admitted for immediate surgery.

Acetylpromazine

Acetylpromazine is an α-antagonist with no significant analgesic properties which causes marked and long-lasting vasodilation, therefore altering blood pressure, CRT, oral mucous membrane colour, pulse strength and heart rate. This removes the patient's ability to use vasoconstriction in an attempt to counteract its state of shock and hypotension. It also causes the intestines to become like a flaccid hosepipe. This drug is thus contraindicated in horses with acute intestinal obstruction. Furthermore, anaesthetizing patients for colic surgery with such iatrogenic hypotension superimposed on a reduced circulatory volume carries considerably more anaesthetic risk.

Although acetylpromazine has been seen to help in some types of ileus by its removal of abnormal sympathetic tone, it should generally be avoided for the above reasons, unless it is a well-hydrated animal experiencing only a mild spasmodic colic.

"IF IN DOUBT, SEND IT"

In practice, no one is expected to know everything about all things, but one is expected to know when to call for help and who to send a case to, without delay. Never hesitate to seek a second opinion. If there is any doubt, the best course of action is to contact an equine referral facility and request that the case be seen at the earliest opportunity. Few in such a facility will object to seeing a suspected surgical colic in good time. Conversely, it is depressing to be on the receiving end of a case of colic caused by a surgical lesion that was either masked by flunixin meglumine or sent too late.

If the patient is insured for veterinary fees and mortality, it would be prudent to contact the insurance company and advise it of the situation and likely need for surgery. If the emergency occurs outside office hours, contact should be made with the office at risk at the earliest opportunity on the next working day to advise it of the state of play.

HOW TO SEND IT

Cost

It is important to explain to the owner that surgical treatment of colic is probably the single most invasive surgical procedure carried out in the horse, and that it is not just a case of opening, curing it, sewing it back together and sending it straight home again. There is also a considerable amount of intensive, all-important and unfortunately expensive aftercare to prevent or relieve ileus and other postoperative complications. Surgical treatment of colic is a high-risk procedure with substantial costs and few guarantees of success.

Final assessment

Just before departure, a final examination should be made to ensure that irreversible metabolic and circulatory changes (deepening cyanosis, coldness of mucous membranes, a heart rate exceeding 100 beats per minute, rectal appreciation of intestinal rupture or severe mental depression) have not developed that might indicate the patient is likely to die in transit, or arrive in a moribund state.

Stomach tube placement

The positive benefit in decompression of the stomach and small intestines far outweighs any temporary ileus resulting from a case with suspected surgical colic travelling with a stomach tube in place. The tube should be secured to the headcollar with tape or to the nostrils with sutures, to prevent it coming out.

Recent history

It is better to send the case with a written account of the clinical findings and all drugs given during the episode than to rely on those involved in the transport to relay accurately all the necessary details. This applies especially to "out of hours" colics – there may not be full transfer of information to the colic team at the time of original telephone contact to arrange the emergency referral.

Directions

It is better for veterinary surgeons to give written copies of maps or directions to the referral facility to clients on their departure in such emergency circumstances, than to depend on them memorizing verbal oral directions.

Telephone contact

It is very helpful for the colic team to know the actual time of departure from the owner's premises and subsequently of any delay in the journey or demise of the patient en route. It is therefore prudent to provide the client with the telephone number of the surgical facility.

Analgesia for transport

It is important to discuss with the surgical team the most appropriate drugs to ensure a comfortable journey for the patient, without complicating the clinical picture of the patient on arrival at the surgical facility.

FURTHER TESTS AT THE SURGICAL FACILITY

Although a variety of specialized tests and equipment can be brought to bear on the presenting acute abdomen, it is the alterations in the findings of the clinical examination of the case that will tell one most about the need for surgery. It is essential to interpret those findings first. Further tests indicate more about the prognosis and therefore whether the surgery is likely to be worthwhile. Such tests may require more sophisticated laboratory or ultrasonographic equipment than is practical in the field and so it is perhaps more appropriate for these extra clinical tools to be applied when the animal reaches the surgical facility.

LABORATORY CLINICAL PATHOLOGY

Laboratory tests are more valuable in deciding the eventual prognosis of the colic case than in the diagnostic decision of the need for surgery. When these tests are correctly applied the client may be better informed of the prognosis and the chances of success with surgery, or of the high likelihood of being left with a "big bill and a dead horse". Owners may still request surgery as a last resort, realizing that they are agreeing more to an expensive method of euthanasia and postmortem, than to a realistic attempt to treat the case surgically.

Tests that can be helpful include complete blood count, total protein and acid-base status, blood lactate, blood urea nitrogen and blood glucose. However, they may be better utilized in the assessment of the degree of cardiovascular compromise and in determining the appropriate medical therapy prior to surgery, than in the decision to operate.

Considerable research is being concentrated on the effect on the normal cardiovascular physiology and the disruption of haemostatic tests by the release of endotoxins. Colics with a thrombocytopenia ($< 50 \times 10^9$/litre), prolonged thrombin time and elevated fibrinogen degradation products ($> 20 \, \text{mg/ml}$) caused by the circulatory shock are considered to carry a very poor prognosis (Fischer, 1989) and may be at extra risk of developing a disseminated intravascular coagulopathy if they survive long enough. It is expected that new and quick tests evaluating the process of haemostasis as a marker of the degree of endotoxic shock will become available in the near future.

Milne *et al.* (1990) evaluated the peritoneal fluid of a variety of cases and noted that medical colics had normal values of white cell count, specific gravity, total protein and alkaline phosphatase activity. Surgical colic cases tended to have sero-sanguineous fluid and a high activity of alkaline phosphatase. Grass sickness cases looked grossly similar to those of medical colics but had a lower specific activity of alkaline phosphatase, a higher total protein content and higher specific gravity than the medical colics. Grass sickness cases had much lower alkaline phosphatase activity than cases with surgical lesions.

RADIOGRAPHY

Hunt (1987) found that radiography was of little value except in oesophageal studies and gastroduodenal obstructions in foals.

Although the technique does not allow demonstration of abdominal detail in adult horses and is not often used, it is possible to diagnose diaphragmatic hernias, enterolithiasis and sand impactions (Fischer, 1989). It does, however, require the use of rare earth/high-speed films and machines capable of generating 150 kV and 250–300 mA. Feed needs to be withheld in adult animals for at least 3 days beforehand and so this technique is restricted to chronic or low-grade colics in foals and small horses. It is important to radiograph the animal from both sides to maximize chances of obtaining diagnostic plates.

ULTRASONOGRAPHY

Echographic examination of the abdomen may be rewarding in the evaluation of the acute abdomen which can be scanned from an external transcutaneous or transrectal approach. Low-

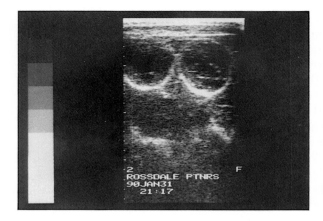

Fig. 5.8 Distended loops of small intestine.

frequency transducers (e.g. 3.5 MHz) are most suitable as they allow maximum depth of penetration (approximately 24 cm). Either sector or linear array transducers can be used. The latter allow more rapid survey scanning, but sector scanners are easier to use between the costal margins.

Ultrasound can be useful in foals, weanlings and ponies where rectal examination is impossible or limited, and in adult horses to examine the cranial region of the abdomen.

Conditions that may be diagnosed include distended loops of small intestine (Fig. 5.8), intussusceptions of the small intestine (Fig. 5.9), caecocaecum and caecocolon (this appears classically as a "doughnut"). Peritoneal fluid is easily visualized, aiding

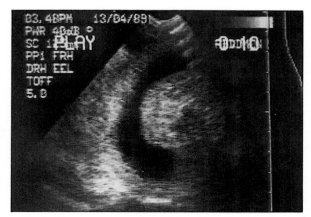

Fig. 5.9 Intussusception of small intestine.

its collection by abdominocentesis. The nature of the fluid can also be assessed by ultrasound and may confirm the presence of fibrinous peritonitis (Fig. 5.10), a ruptured viscus, perforated ulcer or ruptured bladder. The presence of ileus may be identified when the normal rhythmic contractions of bowel and passage of contents through the lumen cannot be visualized over a prolonged period. Loops of bowel that remain static and fixed in location may suggest the presence of adhesions. Abdominal masses may be detected, or transrectal ultrasound may identify the nature of a mass discovered on rectal examination. Visceral displacement may be appreciated, particularly entrapment of the large bowel over the nephrosplenic ligament.

The main disadvantages of ultrasound are that gas-filled bowel and air-filled lung prevent effective imaging beyond these structures, and the restricted depth penetration results in the central core of the abdomen being inaccessible to this technique.

ENDOSCOPY AND LAPAROSCOPY

Alimentary endoscopy is more commonly used to evaluate suspected gastrointestinal ulceration in foals or adults than in acute colics, as it usually requires starvation of the patient for at least 24 hours to minimize the presence of gastric contents.

There are more indications for laparoscopy in cases of chronic colic which have abnormal rectal findings than those in acute pain (Fischer *et al.*, 1986).

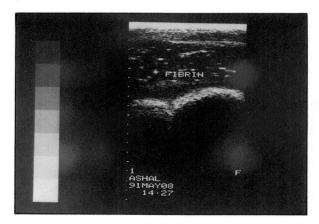

Fig. 5.10 Fibrinous peritonitis.

SUMMARY

A horse in abdominal pain demands a decision without necessarily a specific diagnosis. Diagnostic nuances can be discussed at leisure after the animal has made a recovery and not before it has taken its chance under the knife. Moore (1986) suggested that perhaps it is not the "decision for surgery" that needs to be made, but rather whether it would be prudent to transfer the animal to a facility where surgery would be performed rapidly, if needed. If the answer to that question is "Yes", the case may be best served by a prompt referral to a surgical facility.

There are no easy answers to the problem of diagnosing the surgical colic. No predictive model will be 100% accurate, and clinicians, at whatever stage in the disease course, will always have to compile the diagnostic jigsaw with their clinical instinct, using evidence from certain clinicopathological data and physical examination findings.

Ducharme *et al.* (1983) and Pascoe *et al.* (1983) stated that in their experience between 8% and 24% of horses treated surgically die or are euthanased during surgery because of the advanced state of the disease. If one is unsure, the single most effective action is to explain the costs and send the patient to a facility where there may be greater experience in surgical cases, a well-equipped surgical facility and a competent team. The surgical team will be in a much better position to eliminate cases that do not have a surgical abdominal lesion because of disease progression (deterioration or resolution) and because of the availability of more sophisticated diagnostic tests. Referring veterinary surgeons will be given maximum support by the colic team in all circumstances. However, if there is unnecessary delay in sending a surgical lesion, this may be more difficult.

It is vital to get the patient to the premises before the entrapped intestine has become strangulated and the inevitable vascular compromise has developed. As soon as the intestines require any form of resection, the chances of the patient returning home alive are dramatically reduced. Time is thus especially important in small intestinal obstructions, and the major responsibility for assessing and managing such cases has to depend on the first opinion clinician (Pearson, 1986).

The key to success in colic surgery is being able to make the decision to perform surgery as soon as possible. The owners must be warned early on in the course of the disease about the potential need for surgery. The vital question is not "What is the precise lesion?", but a much more basic "Might this animal need surgical intervention?". If the answer is "Yes", then send it, please don't sit on it.

Acknowledgements

The author wishes to thank A. J. McGladdery for his assistance on the section on abdominal ultrasound and Virginia Reef for her ultrasonogram of a small intestinal intussusception.

REFERENCES AND FURTHER READING

Clark, E. S. & Becht, J. L. (1987) Clinical pharmacology of the gastrointestinal tract. *Veterinary Clinics of North America (Equine Practice)* **3**, 101–122.

Ducharme, N. G., Hackett, R. P. & Ducharme, G. R. (1983) Surgical treatment of colic results in 181 horses. *Veterinary Surgery* **12** (4), 206–209.

Edwards, G. B. (1985) Abdominal surgery. In *Equine Medicine and Surgery 1* (Ed. J. Hickman) pp. 105–193. Academic Press, New York.

Edwards, G. B. (1988) Prognosis in equine colic. *Veterinary Annual* **28**, 102–128.

Edwards, G. B. (1991) Equine colic – the decision for surgery. *Equine Veterinary Education* **3** (1), 19–23.

Fischer, A. T. (1989) Diagnostic and prognostic procedures for equine colic surgery. *Veterinary Clinics of North America (Equine Practice)* **5** (2), 335–348.

Fischer, A. T., Lloyd, K. C. K. & Carlson, G. P. (1986) Diagnostic laparoscopy in the horse. *Journal of the American Veterinary Medical Association* **189**, 289–292.

Hunt, J. (1987) Rectal examination of the equine gastrointestinal tract. *In Practice* **9**, 171–177.

Milne, E. M., Doxey, D. L. & Gilmour, J. S. (1990) Analysis of peritoneal fluid as a diagnostic aid in grass sickness (equine dysautonomia). *Veterinary Record* **127**, 162–165.

Moore, J. N. (1986) *Proceedings of the Veterinary Seminar at the University of Georgia*, Equine acute abdomen. pp. 12–14.

Parry, B. W. (1982) Prognosis and the necessity for surgery in equine colic. *Veterinary Bulletin* **52**, 249–260.

Parry, B. W. (1987) Use of clinical pathology in evaluation of horses with colic. *Veterinary Clinics of North America* **3** (3), 529–542.

Pascoe, P. J., McDonnell, W. N. & Trim, C. M. (1983) Mortality rates and associated factors in equine colic operations – a retrospective study of 341 operations. *Canadian Veterinary Journal* **24**, 76–85.

Pearson, H. (1986) Responsible referral for colic surgery. *Equine Veterinary Journal* **18** (4), 247–248.

Rantanen, N. W. (1986) Diseases of the abdomen. *Veterinary Clinics of North America (Equine Practice)* **2** (1), 67–88.

Rose, E. M. & Rose, J. A. (1988) Initial treatment of colic. *Veterinary Clinics of North America (Equine Practice)* **4**, 35–49.

Stashak, T. S. (1982) Clinical evaluation of the equine colic patient. *Veterinary Clinics of North America (Large Animal Practice)* **1**, 175–288.

Thurmon, J. C. (1990) General considerations for anaesthesia of the horse. *Veterinary Clinics of North America (Equine Practice)* **6** (3), 485–494.

Turner, T. A., Adams, S. B. & White, N. A. (1984) Small intestine incarceration through the epiploic foramen of the horse. *Journal of the American Veterinary Medical Association* **184** (6), 731–734.

Urquhart, K. (1987) Nasogastric intubation of the horse. *In Practice* **9** (3), 84–85.

CHAPTER 6

Investigation and Management of Recurrent Colic

MICHAEL SCHRAMME

Recurrent colic refers to the occurrence of repeated bouts of abdominal discomfort. This definition is vague as it does not specify the duration of the periods of remission, nor the patient's overall condition during these periods. The distinction between recurrent colic and chronic colic, in which pain may wax and wane with variable intensity for more than 48 hours without signs of strangulation, can be difficult and is merely based on the subjective assessment of the attending clinician. In this chapter, recurrent colic is defined as two or more episodes of abdominal pain, separated by a period of remission of at least several days.

CLASSIFICATION

Although evidence of discomfort or abnormal behaviour is sometimes mistaken for colic, colic pain generally emanates from the abdominal cavity. Gastrointestinal disorders obviously top the differential list, but abnormalities of extraintestinal abdominal organs may also generate intermittent abdominal discomfort. Alimentary abdominal pain results from intestinal distension, spasm or ischaemia; it may also be produced by mesenteric tension and the release of inflammatory mediators.

A classification of the causes of recurrent colic, based on their anatomical location and pathogenesis of pain, is outlined below. Of the conditions listed, the most commonly encountered as causes of recurrent colic are:

(1)   Small intestinal stenosis, subtotal obstructions and muscular hypertrophy.
(2)   Large intestinal obstructions.
(3)   Intestinal neoplasia.
(4)   Gastrointestinal parasitism.
(5)   Abdominal abscess.
(6)   Abdominal adhesions.
(7)   Gastroduodenal ulceration and gastric distension.
(8)   Chronic grass sickness.
(9)   Urogenital disorders.
(10) Hepatic disease.

CAUSES OF RECURRENT COLIC

Gastrointestinal causes

Gastric pain

Gastroduodenal ulcer syndrome (Fig. 6.1); pyloric stenosis; aerophagia; mural infiltration (squamous cell carcinoma).

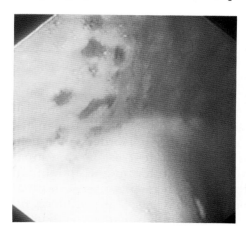

Fig. 6.1 Endoscopic view of a stomach. A peptic ulcer can be observed in the glandular mucosa. The patient presented with a history of intermittent abdominal pain, inappetence and depression (courtesy of D. Knottenbelt).

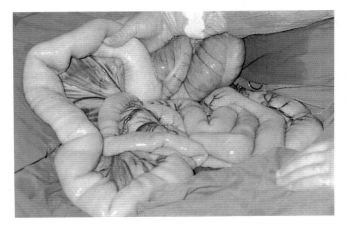

Fig. 6.2 Chronic muscular hypertrophy of the ileum and distal jejunum associated with chronic intermittent colic. Note the thickened, rubbery bowel wall. This has lost its ability to contract to normal size and therefore has a flaccid, folded appearance, even though the bowel lumen is empty.

Intestinal stenosis

(1) *Mural thickening.* Ileal hypertrophy (Fig. 6.2); ileocaecal stenosis; mucosal ulceration (NSAID toxicity); intramural neoplasia: lymphosarcoma (Fig. 6.3), leiomyoma, adenocarcinoma; infiltrative bowel disease (granulomatous, eosinophilic).

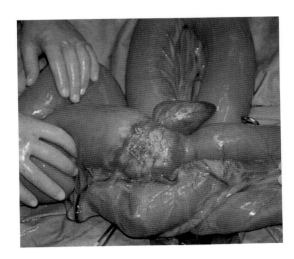

Fig. 6.3 Isolated lymphosarcoma causing a subtotal obstruction of the jejunal lumen. Colic episodes in this patient invariably occurred immediately after feeding, and had become more frequent and pronounced in recent weeks. The condition was treated successfully by resection and anastomosis.

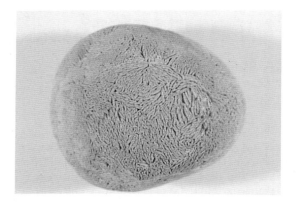

Fig. 6.4 A 9 cm diameter enterolith, associated with recurrent abdominal discomfort.

(2)   *Partial luminal obstruction.* Ileal diverticulum; enterolithiasis (Fig. 6.4); foreign body obstruction; sand impaction.
(3)   *Incomplete displacement or incarceration.* Pedunculated lipoma obstruction; epiploic foramen entrapment; diaphragmatic hernia; intussusception (Figs 6.5, 6.6); adhesion-associated malpositioning.

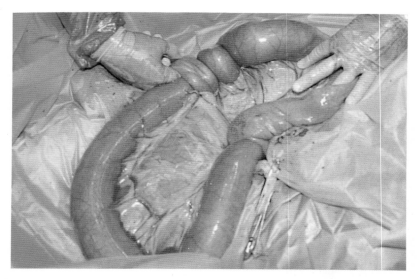

Fig. 6.5 Jejunojejunal intussusception found during laparotomy. The surgeon's index finger enters the intussuscipiens with the intussusceptum.

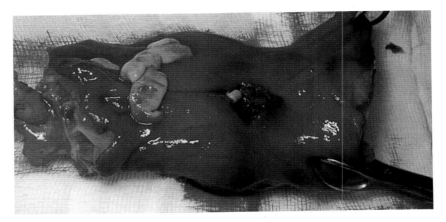

Fig. 6.6 Several tapeworms are present on the mucosal surface of this resected segment of intussuscepted ileum.

Intestinal motility derangement

Management (feeding, dental care, water access); environmental factors (stress, exercise, weather); intestinal parasitism (Fig. 6.7); chronic grass sickness; caecal dysfunction; aerophagia; adhesions (Fig. 6.8).

Peritoneal/mesenteric pain

Localized, chronic peritonitis; mesenteric abscess (Fig. 6.9); adhesions; mesenteric haematoma.

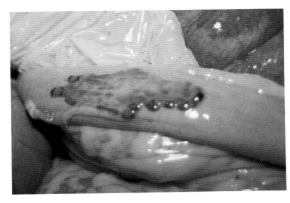

Fig. 6.7 Haemomelasma ilei can be an incidental finding during exploratory laparotomy. Even though these serosal scars have been associated with strongyle migration, their clinical significance is questionable. These lesions do not warrant surgical removal.

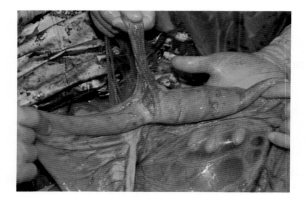

Fig. 6.8 Exploratory laparotomy in a foal with recurrent abdominal pain following small intestinal resection and anastomosis 3 months previously. A firm, singular adhesion connects the omentum to the healed jejunojejunal anastomosis, and causes a partial obstruction. Note the hypertrophy of the jejunum proximal to the site of obstruction (on the palm of the surgeon's right hand).

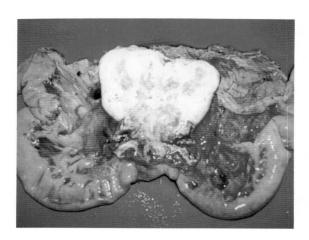

Fig. 6.9 Mesenteric abscess associated with chronic unthriftiness and colic in a yearling. The extensive mesenteric inflammation with adhesion formation restricts normal movement of the involved bowel segment.

Extraintestinal causes

Urogenital disorders

Cystitis; cystic calculi; bladder neoplasia; ovulation pain; granulosa cell tumour; chronic inguinal abscess; testicular teratoma.

Hepatic disorders

Hepatitis; cholelithiasis; cholangitis.

Splenic disorders

Splenic tumours; splenomegaly; splenic displacement (nephrosplenic entrapment).

Pancreas disorders

Pancreatitis?

CLINICAL INVESTIGATION

The initial clinical assessment of a patient with a history of recurrent abdominal discomfort is not dissimilar to the diagnostic work-up for an animal with an acute abdominal crisis (Table 6.1). Since the patient will generally be experiencing one of its recurrent bouts of pain at the time of presentation, the clinician's first concern should be to establish whether or not it requires emergency surgery in order to survive; this will

Table 6.1 Investigative options for the diagnostic work-up of patients with recurrent abdominal pain.

History	**Biopsy techniques**
General appearance and accompanying signs	Intestinal biopsy
	Ileal biopsy in grass sickness
	Lymph node biopsy
Clinical examination	Rectal biopsy
Cardiovascular parameters	Liver biopsy
Rectal palpation	
Abdominocentesis	**Diagnostic/therapeutic treatment**
	Dental care
Laboratory clinical pathology	Anthelmintics
Haematology and biochemistry	Spasmolytics
Liver function test	Corticosteroids
Monosaccharide absorption test	Prokinetics
Faecal analysis	
	Exploratory laparotomy
Imaging techniques	
Endoscopy	
Radiography	
Ultrasonography	
Laparoscopy	

involve a step-by-step assessment of the patient, paying particular attention to the cardiovascular and gastrointestinal systems. When it has been ascertained that there is no immediate life-threatening problem, sufficient time will be available to expand on the preliminary clinical information by repeating certain investigations, extending them to include different body systems, laboratory analysis or imaging techniques.

The presenting signs of patients with intermittent colic may vary considerably. Colic may be an isolated clinical sign in an otherwise healthy individual, or may be accompanied by diarrhoea, weight loss and signs of generalized systemic disease (Fig. 6.10). In the latter case, colic is rarely the reason for seeking veterinary assistance. For a discussion of the syndromes of chronic diarrhoea, weight loss and hepatic disease the reader is referred to O'Brien (1985), Brown (1989), Milne (1990) and Love (1992).

No matter how extensive the work-up, attempts to diagnose specific causes of recurrent abdominal discomfort can be very difficult, expensive and, ultimately, unrewarding. In a number of patients a diagnostic exploratory laparotomy may be resorted to, but even this may be unsuccessful.

HISTORY

Onset and duration of the problem, frequency of recurrence and time interval between bouts of colic

An increasing frequency of recurrence of colic with a shorter time interval between bouts may indicate a progressively

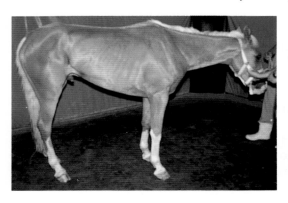

Fig. 6.10 A wasting horse with chronic weight loss, inappetence and diarrhoea may present with a history of recurrent abdominal discomfort.

worsening compromise to the bowel lumen. Abdominal pain that waxes and wanes in relation to feeding may indicate the presence of a partial obstruction of the proximal intestine (e.g. neoplasia, muscular hypertrophy or gastric ulcer). Regular 3-week intervals between colic bouts in mares can be related to ovulation pain.

Previous medical history

Previous abdominal surgery or injury predisposes to adhesion formation. A history of respiratory disease or septicaemia should alert the examiner to the possibility of abdominal abscesses, while long-term medication with non-steroidal anti-inflammatory drugs (NSAIDs) is a risk factor for gastrointestinal ulceration.

Age and type of patient

Young foals and yearlings are prone to gastric ulceration, intussusceptions and foreign body obstructions, while aged individuals are more likely candidates for neoplasia and dysfunction of caecal or colonic motility. Aged ponies are particularly susceptible to pedunculated lipoma obstructions.

Individual horse or herd problem

The occurrence of recurrent abdominal discomfort in several horses belonging to the same herd or stables should prompt detailed questioning on management and environmental factors. It may be important not merely to discuss management techniques, but to make a farm visit to investigate them on-site.

Environmental and management factors

Management, including water access and quality, should be closely inspected. Rations excessively high in carbohydrates can result from overfeeding grain, group feeding allowing aggressive horses to overeat, or from providing inadequate quantities of roughage. These practices predispose to the development of an atypical intestinal microflora and may lead to diarrhoea, excessive gas production, derangement of intestinal motility and colic. Similar complications may result from sudden changes in feeding pattern or irregular time intervals between feeding.

Poor quality roughage, mouldy hay or an inadequate water supply can predispose animals to simple colonic impactions. Investigation of the horse's environment should include an assessment of the quantity and quality of stable bedding and examination for any evidence of crib biting. Sandy pastures and starvation paddocks may lead to sand colic, especially if animals are fed from the ground.

Two other vital components of good preventive management are parasite control and regular dental care.

The neonatal management routine in breeding farms should be assessed in view of the incidence of gastroduodenal ulcer syndrome.

GENERAL APPEARANCE AND ACCOMPANYING SIGNS

The clinical signs of abdominal discomfort may be accompanied by other abnormalities that may guide the preliminary diagnosis: patients with diarrhoea and weight loss may be suffering from enteritis, malabsorption or infiltration of the bowel wall by a neoplastic or inflammatory process; jaundice or nervous signs may indicate involvement of the liver; dysuria or haematuria are present when cystitis or cystic calculi are the initiating cause of discomfort; intermittent or persistent fever is likely to reflect a systemic infection, abdominal abscess or peritonitis.

CLINICAL EXAMINATION

The clinical examination protocol is identical to that used in any case of colic, in concentrating initially on the cardiovascular system and gastrointestinal function. Deterioration of cardiovascular parameters, although rare in recurrent colic, may indicate significant dehydration or compromised bowel wall viability.

Rectal palpation

Rectal palpation is probably the procedure most likely to produce a positive finding in cases of recurrent colic. The clinician should, therefore, take sufficient time to perform a meticulous and thorough examination, if necessary at full arm's length. Fractious or straining patients are best medicated with sedative or spasmolytic drugs to facilitate the procedure and allow the time necessary for thorough but safe palpation. At a dose rate of 0.6–1 mg/kg, the sedative effect of intravenous xylazine lasts for approximately 20 minutes. Intravenous injection of 0.2 mg/kg propantheline bromide or 0.15–0.20 mg/kg hyoscine N-butylbromide causes a profound relaxation of the rectum within minutes.

The best time to perform a rectal palpation is during an actual episode of abdominal pain. Nevertheless, the examination should be repeated when the pain has subsided, to compare the rectal pictures; often abnormalities can only be felt when signs of pain are displayed by the patient. Even though a large number of animals with recurrent colic will present with a normal rectal picture, there are some specific rectal findings that should be looked for in these patients (Table 6.2).

Muscular hypertrophy of the small intestine will be recognized by palpation of a thick and rubbery bowel wall. The bowel has often lost its ability to contract to normal size, and feels like deflated or inflated bicycle inner tubing, depending on the absence or presence of intestinal distension. Hypertrophy tends to occur first at the level of the ileum and may extend in an oral direction in chronic cases. These changes either reflect or form a long-standing partial obstruction of the bowel lumen and are an indication for exploratory surgery.

Distension of the small intestine is recognized by the palpation of gas-filled loops (sometimes compared to sausage rings) in the central abdomen. Severe distension, characteristic of acute and complete obstruction, with a tense bowel wall is uncommon in recurrent colic. Moderate distension, with abnormally obvious but still indentable loops of bowel, is more characteristic of the transient distension that often accompanies recurrent colic. It may reflect the presence of a partial obstruction or intermittent partial ileus. These changes often occur in relation to feeding, and are most obvious on palpation during an episode of pain. Often the abdomen feels completely normal during

Table 6.2 Detectability of various causes of recurrent colic by rectal examination.

COMMONLY DETECTABLE

Thickening of the intestinal wall
Chronic small intestinal stenosis, ileal hypertrophy, ileocaecal stenosis, intramural neoplasia (lymphosarcoma, leiomyoma, adenocarcinoma), infiltrative bowel disease (granulomatous, eosinophilic)

Small intestinal distension
Small intestinal stenosis, ileal diverticulum, pedunculated lipoma obstruction, subtotal epiploic foramen entrapment, intussusception, adhesion-associated malpositioning

Small intestinal spasm
Intestinal parasitism, ischaemic bowel disease, recurrent bowel irritation

Large intestinal distension
Enterolithiasis, foreign body obstruction, sand impaction, diaphragmatic hernia, caecal dysfunction

Presence of a palpable mass
Mesenteric abscess, cystitis, bladder neoplasia, cystic calculi, ovulation, granulosa cell tumour, chronic inguinal abscess, testicular teratoma, splenic tumours (lymphosarcoma), splenomegaly

COMMONLY UNDETECTABLE

Hepatitis, cholelithiasis, cholangitis
Chronic pancreatitis
Gastroduodenal ulcer syndrome, pyloric stenosis, aerophagia, gastric mural infiltration (squamous cell carcinoma)
Mucosal ulceration (NSAID toxicity)

VARIABLE DETECTABILITY

Intestinal parasitism
Chronic grass sickness
Localized, chronic peritonitis
Adhesions
Mesenteric haematoma
Diaphragmatic hernia
Intramural neoplasia

periods of remission from pain, illustrating the importance of these findings.

A *palpable abdominal mass* is always an alarming finding. Its consistency may be rock-hard (in the case of an enterolith), fleshy to firm (neoplasm, intussusception or inguinal abscess), indentable (impaction) or fluctuating (haematoma of the broad ligament). Careful palpation should enable the clinician to identify tentatively the location of the mass in relation to the abdominal organs: impactions and intussusceptions will be located in the bowel lumen, alimentary lymphosarcoma in the intestinal wall, abscesses in the mesentery, calculi within the bladder, and neoplasia within the spleen, kidney or ovary. Occasionally, adhesions can be identified by localized 'knotting' of the mesentery with a fixed, intermittently distended loop of bowel. Such an area of localized chronic inflammation within the mesentery or on the peritoneal surface may also give the impression of an abdominal mass.

Small intestinal hyperperistalsis may be felt during recurrent episodes of abdominal pain as intermittent waves of exaggerated peristalsis. The violent bowel spasms are identified by the quickly changing diameter of bowel segments, which may contract to pencil size during severe spasm and relax immediately afterwards.

Abdominocentesis

Peritoneal fluid can be obtained by needle abdominocentesis (see Chapter 5) or with a teat cannula. With the former technique, the risk of damaging the intestinal wall is real, and even though a small hole in the bowel wall usually seals over quickly in healthy bowel, this procedure should not be undertaken lightly. In one report, the incidence of enterocentesis in horses with colic was 6%, with two horses developing peritonitis and one horse abdominal wall cellulitis (Siex and Wilson, 1992); the author has seen similar complications, some with fatal consequences. The use of a teat cannula is slightly more invasive and requires a strictly aseptic technique. However, the strike rate is higher and there is less risk of enterocentesis.

Complications are more likely to arise from abdominocentesis in cases where there is distended bowel; a gravid uterus; sand in the colon weighing down the bowel; fibrous adhesions between the large bowel and body wall; or devitalized bowel in the ventral abdomen. A rectal examination should, therefore, be performed prior to abdominocentesis. Recognition of any of these conditions may be a reason to omit this procedure if it is not vitally important for the diagnosis.

The analysis of peritoneal fluid is a sensitive indicator of bowel injury and/or peritoneal inflammation (Table 6.3). In recurrent colic patients, however, the results of peritoneal fluid analysis are frequently within normal limits. Any aberrations are often limited to unspecific signs of inflammation of the visceral or parietal peritoneum, reflected by a variable rise in leucocytes and the protein level. Red blood cell leakage from the capillaries in the intestinal wall with serosanguineous discoloration of the peritoneal fluid is rare, since devitalization of bowel is not a common feature of recurrent colic.

Some particular abnormalities of the fluid have been associated with specific causes of recurrent abdominal discomfort as described below, although these changes are often inconsistent and some of them are found, at best, only in exceptional cases.

(1) In simple bowel obstructions, a slow increase in the protein level of peritoneal fluid is seen, with no concurrent rise in red or white blood cells. In the absence of ischaemic bowel, the neutrophil/macrophage ratio should remain normal.
(2) In sand impactions, sand may be obtained if the bowel is perforated during abdominocentesis.
(3) In intussusceptions, fluid changes may often not reflect the severity of bowel wall compromise. As bowel wall compromise progresses, the peritoneal fluid should become more serosanguineous, with a more significant elevation in leucocytes and the protein level. However, the compromised intussusceptum may be contained within the less compromised intussuscipiens, preventing bowel leakage directly into the peritoneal cavity.
(4) In non-strangulating infarctions due to intestinal parasitism, peritoneal fluid changes usually reflect a degree of peritonitis. Red blood cells are present in about 50% of cases. An increased number of eosinophils ($> 5\%$) has been interpreted as suggestive of, but not pathognomonic for, this condition.
(5) In abdominal neoplasia, peritoneal fluid changes are difficult to differentiate from other inflammatory conditions. Exfoliated tumour cells are a possible but rare finding.

LABORATORY CLINICAL PATHOLOGY

Haematology and biochemistry

In cases of recurrent colic, unlike the acute abdomen, time is available to obtain a complete haematological and biochemical

Table 6.3 Peritoneal fluid changes associated with some causes of recurrent colic.

	Colour	Turbidity	Erythrocytes	Leucocytes ($\times 10^9$/litre)	Protein (g/litre)	Cytology
Normal	Pale yellow	Clear	–	5–8	<25	Neutrophil: macrophage ratio 2:1
Simple obstruction	Pale yellow	Clear	–	5–8	25–35	2:1
Grass sickness	Yellow	Clear	–	5–8	>30	2:1
Enteritis	Yellow	Clear	–	Slightly raised	>30	2:1
Peritonitis	Serosanguineous	Turbid	Variable	>100	35–65	>2:1 Degenerate neutrophils Bacteria possible
Non-strangulating infarction	This condition can mimic any other type of peritoneal fluid response, including increases in erythrocytes, leucocytes and total protein					

profile. Often, clinicopathological findings are within normal limits, or consistent with non-specific low-grade chronic inflammation or intestinal obstruction. However, some alterations may be associated with selected conditions, as follows.

With abdominal abscess formation, plasma protein, fibrinogen and gamma-globulin levels are often elevated, while albumin concentration is normal or decreased.

In verminous arteritis, laboratory findings vary greatly from normal to mild inflammation. Eosinophilia is commonly associated with parasite infiltration, and serum electrophoresis has been used to identify a β_2-globulin peak associated with larval migration. However, neither parameter is specific for parasite problems or *Strongylus vulgaris* larvae migration.

Foals with gastric ulceration can be anaemic and hypoproteinaemic. Duodenal ulceration may be accompanied by evidence of ascending cholangitis and hepatitis (elevated levels of gamma-glutamyl transferase, alkaline phosphatase and serum bile acids). However, these enzyme levels may also occur in foals with obstructive bowel disease without occlusive liver disease.

In rare cases of lymphosarcoma, leukaemia may be present with a leucocyte count of $40–80 \times 10^9$/litre, and a differential increase in lymphocytes. Hypercalcaemia is another rare finding. Abnormal lymphocytes may be seen in the peripheral circulation. Hypergammaglobulinaemia may be present. Other signs of chronic inflammation, such as anaemia and hyperfibrinogenaemia, are generally not present.

Clinicopathological changes of chronic NSAID toxicity often include hypoproteinaemia, haemoconcentration, elevation in blood urea nitrogen and creatinine values, and variable leucocyte counts and electrolyte imbalances.

Hypoproteinaemia and hypoalbuminaemia in granulomatous and eosinophilic gastroenteritis, as well as other infiltrative bowel diseases, reflect a protein-losing enteropathy.

Laboratory data in hepatic disease include low blood urea nitrogen, high or normal serum globulins, and elevated bilirubin, bile acids and liver enzymes, and are reviewed elsewhere (Milne, 1990).

Liver function tests

Bromsulphalein (BSP) clearance and bile acid assay have been used as liver function tests (Milne, 1990).

Monosaccharide absorption tests

The rate and extent of absorption of glucose or D-xylose from the small intestine may be reduced in horses with chronic colic, accompanied by signs of chronic weight loss and/or diarrhoea. This reduction may be due to delayed gastric emptying, infiltrative bowel diseases (neoplasia) or reduced bowel perfusion secondary to parasitic damage.

Faecal analysis

Faecal examination should include gross, cytological and bacteriological evaluations. The efficiency of mastication or colonic transit time is reflected in the faecal consistency or particle size. The presence of sand is often not palpable in the faeces but can be identified in the sediment (a faecal sample and water are placed in a rectal sleeve which is left hanging vertically to allow sedimentation). Qualitative examinations for worm eggs can be performed for the most common equine intestinal parasites, large and small strongyles, tapeworms and roundworms (DiPietro, 1992; Proudman, 1994). Faecal egg counts are of limited diagnostic value in strongylid infections, since larvae, rather than egg-laying adults, are responsible for the verminous arteritis and ischaemic bowel changes. However, they may give an indication of the general efficiency of the parasite control programme for the patient in question.

Faecal occult blood has been associated with gastroduodenal ulceration and NSAID toxicity. The test is of limited diagnostic value, however, as both false negative and false positive results have been documented. Faecal culture techniques are designed to isolate *Salmonella* species in patients with recurrent colic and accompanying chronic or intermittent diarrhoea. Recovery of this organism is diagnostic, although it may also be recovered in patients that are asymptomatic carriers.

IMAGING TECHNIQUES

A variety of advanced imaging techniques can be used in the investigation of the horse's abdomen. These include endoscopy, ultrasonography, radiography and laparoscopy.

Endoscopy

Alimentary endoscopy is used almost exclusively to evaluate the presence of gastroduodenal ulceration or squamous cell carcinoma as possible primary causes of colic. The nasal passages of foals will only allow the insertion of endoscopes with an outer diameter of 10 mm or less; larger diameter endoscopes can only be used in adults. An insertion tube length of 200 cm or more is required to reach the stomach of adult horses; for young foals (30 days), 110 cm will suffice, while for weanlings, a length of up to 180 cm is needed.

In foals, the majority of ulcerations are seen in the non-glandular mucosa, especially adjacent to the margo plicatus; these foals are often asymptomatic. Lesions of the glandular mucosa or duodenum are more commonly associated with signs of colic, bruxism and interrupted nursing. Lesions around the pylorus or duodenum may be associated with signs of gastric reflux. Most lesions in yearlings are confined to the squamous mucosa adjacent to the margo plicatus and have been associated with recurrent colic and poor bodily condition. Gastric ulceration is common in adult horses and likewise occurs most frequently in the squamous mucosa adjacent to the margo plicatus. Ulceration associated with NSAID toxicity is often located in the glandular mucosa.

Ultrasonography

Transabdominal wall ultrasonography is particularly useful in animals that do not allow rectal palpation or where the abnormality lies outside rectal reach within the abdomen. Owing to the limited range of penetration, only structures within 25 cm of the abdominal wall can be visualized. In the investigation of the recurrent colic patient, the following signs may be significant.

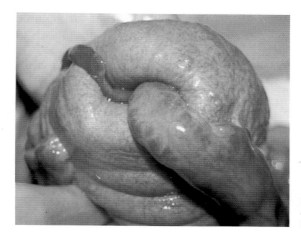

Fig. 6.11 Inversion of the caecal apex in a caecocaecal intussusception in a yearling.

(1)   Ileus and small intestinal distension are characterized by the appearance of distended loops of bowel with static luminal contents. The absence of rhythmic intestinal contractions is indicative of ileus.

(2)   Intussusceptions produce a typical doughnut-like appearance on transverse section (Figs 6.11, 6.12). Such images allow an accurate early diagnosis before irreversible bowel wall degeneration results in deterioration of clinical parameters.

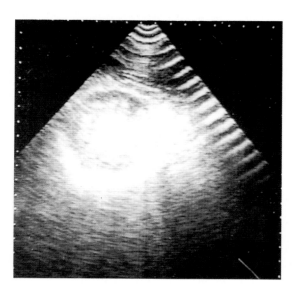

Fig. 6.12 Ultrasonogram, obtained over the ventral body wall, shows the typical doughnut-like appearance of the intussusception in cross-section. The condition was treated successfully by resection.

(3)   Adhesions may be recognized by the fact that an isolated bowel segment does not move relative to adjacent intestines or body wall.

(4)   Increased bowel wall thickness may be observed in cases of muscular hypertrophy of the small intestine.

(5)   The ultrasonographic appearance of abdominal masses may provide information on the nature and structure of the mass and help in differentiating between an abscess and neoplasia. When the ultrasonographic findings do not provide a definitive diagnosis, the use of ultrasound-guided paracentesis or needle biopsy often allows a cytological or histological diagnosis to be reached (Hillyer, 1994).

(6)   The appearance of an enlarged mesenteric root and lesions associated with the cranial mesenteric arteries may indicate the severity of luminal compromise and arterial patency.

(7)   An 88% accuracy in the ultrasonographic diagnosis of entrapment of the left colon in the nephrosplenic space was reported by Santschi et al. (1993). Positive findings were a gas echo obliterating visualization of the dorsal outline of the splenic margin, the image of the left colon lateral to the spleen and ventral displacement of the spleen.

Radiography

Specific causes of recurrent colic which have been diagnosed by radiography are enterolithiasis, cystic calculi, sand impaction of the large colon and chronic diaphragmatic hernia (Fischer, 1989). Gastroduodenal ulceration in foals has been characterized by gastric distension, the presence of air in the hepatic ducts and delayed gastric emptying of contrast (more than 2 hours for complete emptying). Ulcers may be demonstrated as lucent filling defects. The procedure is described by Butler et al. (1993).

Laparoscopy

Indications for laparoscopy in the recurrent colic patient are characterization and biopsy of palpable abdominal masses, investigation of suspected adhesions and examination of the urogenital tract within the pelvic inlet. The technique is described by Fischer *et al.* (1986).

BIOPSY TECHNIQUES

Alimentary tract biopsies are generally obtained for histological and bacteriological examination. Full-thickness bowel specimens provide the most information but require a laparotomy. Smaller samples, taken using endoscopic techniques, are easier to obtain but may provide only limited information.

Intestinal biopsy

Laparotomy under general anaesthesia is commonly the preferred method for obtaining intestinal biopsies, as laparoscopy is not generally available. A full-thickness wedge of bowel is removed from the antimesenteric border in two or three different locations along the intestinal tract where lesions are macroscopically evident. The resulting defect is sutured transversely with a double layer inverting suture pattern. In patients with granulomatous or eosinophilic enteritis or alimentary lymphosarcoma, the biopsy will show diffuse or focal cellular infiltration of the involved cell type.

Ileal biopsy in grass sickness

A technique for ante-mortem diagnosis of grass sickness was described by Scholes *et al.* (1993). During laparotomy, an elliptical piece of ileum, 15 × 10 mm, is excised at the proximal end of the ileocaecal fold, halfway between the mesenteric and antimesenteric borders. The degeneration or complete loss of enteric neurons is diagnostic of grass sickness. In chronic cases, associated with intermittent abdominal pain, the degenerative changes appear to be limited to the distal small intestine. Prior to the development of the ileal biopsy technique, the characteristic neuronal degeneration of the autonomic ganglia, removed within 2 hours of death, was considered the only positive confirmation for a diagnosis of grass sickness.

Lymph node biopsy

The intestinal lymph nodes are localized near the root of the mesentery. Enlarged lymph nodes can be bluntly dissected from the mesentery, or a biopsy instrument can be used to obtain a tissue sample.

Rectal biopsy

Pinch biopsies of the rectal mucosa are obtained with mare uterine biopsy forceps. One of the examiner's hands fixes a fold of ventral rectal mucosa about 30 cm in from the anal spincter. The biopsy forceps are then introduced and guided onto the fold with the other hand. Although the reliability of alterations in rectal tissue has been questioned, histology may reveal foci of cellular infiltration in patients with infiltrative (granulomatous, eosinophilic or lymphosarcomatous) or inflammatory bowel diseases. Bacteriological examination of rectal biopsies has been claimed to enhance the recovery of *Salmonella* species over faecal culture.

In a recent study 52% of patients with clinical signs of intestinal disease had pathological changes in rectal biopsy specimens. Eosinophilic gastroenteritis and granulomatous enteritis were diagnosed from biopsy specimens in 10 of 21 cases (Lindberg *et al.*, 1996).

Liver biopsy

Histological examination of liver tissue can provide a definitive diagnosis in patients with diffuse liver pathology (fibrosis, ragwort poisoning, neoplasia or fatty degeneration); focal lesions, on the other hand, can be easily missed using this technique. The procedure for liver biopsy has been detailed by Milne (1990).

EXPLORATORY LAPAROTOMY

Even though the list of investigative options for the diagnostic work-up of patients with recurrent abdominal pain is exhaustive, the majority of cases will end up undergoing a laparotomy for diagnostic or therapeutic purposes, often in a final attempt to characterize the nature and extent of the abdominal lesion. An exploratory laparotomy allows macroscopic evaluation of the gastrointestinal tract and the biopsy of suspected tissues for histopathological examination.

MANAGEMENT

The therapeutic approach to a patient with recurrent abdominal discomfort can be subdivided into managemental corrections, medical treatment and surgical intervention.

MANAGEMENT CORRECTIONS

Management considerations concern feeding methods, environmental factors, parasite control and dental care.

Feeding methods

One of the most important measures in minimizing the incidence of colic at horse establishments is the enforcement of a regular and individual feeding regimen comprising a balanced ration and adequate fresh water. One of the primary goals is maintaining a stable environment for the bacterial flora of the digestive tract. A few simple tips for avoiding colic are listed below.

(1)   Horses should not be overfed with high concentrate feeds. No more than 2.25 kg (5 lb) of grain should be given in a single meal.
(2)   High concentrate meals should be avoided immediately after exercise.
(3)   A number of small meals is preferable to one or two large meals if the horse is on a high concentrate diet.
(4)   Alternative sources of energy, such as fat and beet pulp, are less likely to cause gastrointestinal upset than unprocessed starch.

(5)   Plenty of fibre should be provided, i.e. a minimum of 1 kg of forage per 100 kg bodyweight per day.
(6)   Bulk laxatives such as bran, psyllium or methylcellulose can be added to the diet of patients with recurrent impactions.
(7)   Food additives such as live yeast cultures or probiotics may be beneficial by stabilizing fermentation in the large bowel.

Environment

Attention should be paid to environmental factors in the management of recurrent colic, as follows:

(1)   Horses kept on sandy pasture should be fed from elevated, clean surfaces.
(2)   All foreign materials (twine, plastic, rubber, etc.) should be removed from the feed and environment.
(3)   Horses that eat their bedding should be bedded on paper clippings or rubber mats.
(4)   Enforced box confinement should be kept to a minimum.
(5)   Stable vices such as aerophagia should be dealt with (e.g. by fitting a neckstrap).

Parasite control

The aim of parasite prophylaxis is to minimize contamination with infective larvae. Current options for the control of equine intestinal parasites are pasture management and anthelmintic drug administration. For practical management guidelines, the reader is referred to Love (1992). The broad-spectrum anthelmintics currently employed are pyrantel salts, benzimidazoles and ivermectin. These drugs should be used in 'slow rotation' to slow down the development of anthelmintic resistance, i.e. the same chemical class should be used for at least a year after which a different chemical class should be instituted each year. Regular analysis of the faecal worm egg count is imperative in order to monitor the efficacy of the programme, especially in view of the high prevalence of benzimidazole resistance.
    Effective tapeworm control can only be achieved with pyrantel embonate (Strongid-P, Pfizer) at twice the antinematode dose (38 mg/kg). This should be undertaken every 6

months, with one treatment in the autumn following summer turnout on pasture.

Dental care

The objective of routine dental prophylaxis is to maintain normal dental occlusion between the lower and upper arcades. Irregular wear, periodontal disease and poor mastication may be responsible for recurrent problems with intestinal impactions. Dental examination and floating should be performed once every 6 months to prevent these problems.

MEDICAL TREATMENT

Gastroduodenal ulceration

Acid-suppressive therapy with H_2-receptor antagonists is effective in healing ulcers and resolving clinical signs in the majority of patients with gastroduodenal ulceration. The currently recommended treatment regimen consists of oral ranitidine (Zantac, Glaxo) at 6.6 mg/kg every 8 hours for a duration of 3 weeks. To ensure complete healing of the lesions, horses should be taken out of training during treatment.

Antacid drugs (aluminium hydroxide or magnesium hydroxide antacids) may also be effective in the treatment of this syndrome, and have been administered at a dosage of 250 ml three times daily to adult horses to prevent the recurrence of gastric ulcers following successful treatment with ranitidine. Sucralfate, a mucosal protectant, may be used as an adjunct to ranitidine treatment at a rate of 2–4 g two to four times daily. Its efficacy in the treatment of equine gastroduodenal ulceration remains undetermined, however.

Spasmolytic and analgesic medication

Recurrent bouts of abdominal discomfort are not unusual following previous colic surgery. Whether these episodes are related to the adverse effects of abdominal adhesions on ingesta flow remains unclear. Clinical experience has shown, however, that a single administration of a spasmolytic or analgesic drug such as hyoscine N-butylbromide and dipyrone (0.2 mg/kg and 25 mg/kg), flunixin meglumine (1.1 mg/kg) or even phenylbutazone (4.4 mg/kg) very often controls such episodes effectively. Occasionally, such an event may lead to an acute abdominal crisis, in which case medication has no – or only a temporary – effect on the pain.

Antibiotic medication for abdominal abscess or peritonitis

Long-term antibiotic cover (up to 6 months) is the recommended medical approach for abdominal abscesses or peritonitis. The oral administration of potassium iodide may also be beneficial in these cases.

Ideally, antibiotic selection should be based on culture and sensitivity test results. Long-term penicillin treatment has been recommended for abdominal abscesses, since the major pathogens involved have often appeared to be sensitive. Peritonitis, on the other hand, is typically multibacterial and the inclusion of an aminoglycoside (gentamicin or amikacin) may also be indicated. Rifampicin (10–20 mg/kg) is often added to the therapeutic regimen because it has the ability to penetrate and help other antibiotics penetrate into abscesses. Metronidazole (20 mg/kg twice daily) may prove effective where *Bacteroides fragilis* is involved.

Symptomatic medication with corticosteroids

In patients with infiltrative bowel disease, in which recurrent abdominal discomfort may be one of the many signs of malabsorption syndrome, successful symptomatic treatment with prednisolone or dexamethasone has been described (Brown, 1989). Patients with alimentary lymphosarcoma have a hopeless prognosis despite an initial favourable response. In other, non-neoplastic, bowel infiltrations, however, this regimen may be successful.

Prokinetic drugs in chronic grass sickness

Recent claims have been made concerning the successful use of the prokinetic drug cisapride (Prepulsid, Janssen-Cilag) in cases of chronic grass sickness (Milne, 1997). The drug can be given orally at 0.8 mg/kg every 8 hours for the first 7 days of treatment. However, in none of the animals studied was a definitive histological diagnosis of grass sickness made. Since an almost total segmental loss of enteric neurons is observed in grass sickness, and these neurons are end-stage cells that cannot be replaced, recovery from this disease would appear to be impossible.

SURGICAL INTERVENTION

The reasons for performing a laparotomy may be a specific diagnosis, the lack of any diagnosis, patient deterioration or lack of improvement with conservative management. (The standard technique of laparotomy and the protocol for abdominal exploration in the horse are widely accepted and have been described extensively.) Euthanasia may be prompted by the macroscopic findings, or a decision may be postponed until information from biopsy samples is available.

Correctable lesions are reduced by the standard surgical techniques of resection and anastomosis. The options available to the surgeon for the surgically correctable causes of recurrent colic are summarized in Table 6.4.

PROGNOSIS OF RECURRENT COLIC

In a recent retrospective study, Mair and Hillyer (1995) found the frequency of episodes of colic to be an important prognostic factor in recurrent transient (each episode of colic lasts less than 24 hours) colic. In a group of 15 horses in which colic occurred 3 times in one month, the main causes were small intestinal obstruction, parasitism or intestinal lymphosarcoma, and the survival rate was 53%. In a group of 27 horses where colic occurred 3 times in one year, the majority of cases suffered spasmodic colic of unknown etiology. The survival rate in the low incidence group was 96%.

Table 6.4 Surgical options.

GASTROINTESTINAL PROCEDURES

Gastroduodenostomy or gastrojejunostomy
Gastroduodenal ulcer syndrome, pyloric stenosis

Ileocaecostomy or jejunocaecostomy without resection of distal segment
Ileal hypertrophy, ileocaecal stenosis

Reduction, resection and jejunojejunostomy or jejunocaecostomy
Isolated intramural neoplasia, ileal diverticulum, foreign body obstruction, pedunculated lipoma obstruction, subtotal epiploic foramen entrapment, intestinal parasitism (ischaemic bowel disease), intussusception, adhesion-associated malpositioning

Side-to-side anastomosis of proximal and distal segment without resection
Adhesion-associated malpositioning

Ileocolostomy or jejunocolostomy
Caecal dysfunction

Large bowel enterotomy and decompression
Enterolithiasis, foreign body obstruction, sand impaction

NON-GASTROINTESTINAL ABDOMINAL PROCEDURES

Reduction and herniorrhaphy
Diaphragmatic hernia

Marsupialization, surgical drainage
Mesenteric abscess, chronic inguinal abscess

Ovariectomy
Ovulation pain, granulosa cell tumour

Cystotomy
Cystic calculus

Splenectomy
Splenic tumours, splenomegaly

Cholelithotripsy or choledochotomy
Cholelithiasis

Laparotomy and castration
Testicular teratoma

EXTRA-ABDOMINAL PROCEDURES

Modified Forssell's procedure
Aerophagia

Acknowledgement

The author wishes to thank Peter Webbon for advice.

REFERENCES AND FURTHER READING

Brown, C. M. (1989) Chronic or recurrent abdominal pain. In *Problems in Equine Medicine* (ed. C. M. Brown) pp. 59–66. Lea & Febiger, Philadelphia.

Butler, J. A., Colles, C. M., Dyson, S. J., Kold, S. E. & Poulos, P. W. (1993) *Clinical Radiology of the Horse*, p. 498. Blackwell Scientific Publications, Oxford.

DiPietro, J. A. (1992) Internal parasite control programs. In *Current Therapy in Equine Medicine*, 3rd edn. (ed. N. E. Robinson) pp. 51–55. W. B. Saunders, Philadelphia.

Fischer, A. T. (1989) Diagnostic and prognostic procedures for equine colic surgery. *Veterinary Clinics of North America* **5**, 335–350.

Fischer, A. T., Lloyd, K. C. & Carlson, G. P. (1986) Diagnostic laparoscopy in the horse. *Journal of the American Veterinary Medical Association* **189**, 289–292.

Hillyer, M. H. (1994) The use of ultrasonography in the diagnosis of abdominal tumours in the horse. *Equine Veterinary Education* **6**, 273–278.

Lindberg, R., Nygren Annica and Persson, S. G. B. (1996) Rectal biopsy in horses with clinical signs of intestinal disorders: a retrospective study of 116 cases. *Equine Veterinary Journal* **28**, 275–284.

Love, S. (1992) The role of equine strongyles in the pathogenesis of colic and current options for prophylaxis. *Equine Veterinary Journal* (supplement) **13**, 5–9.

Mair, T. S. (1995) Recurrent colic. BEVA Specialist Seminar on Equine Abdominal Medicine and Surgery, Sutton Coldfield, 28th April 1995.

Milne, E. M. (1990) Differential diagnosis of hepatic disorders in horses. *In Practice* **12**, 252–258.

Milne, E. M. (1997) Grass sickness: an update. *In Practice* **19**, 128–133.

Milne, E. M., Woodman, M. P. & Doxey, D. L. (1994) Use of clinical measurements to predict the outcome in chronic cases of grass sickness (equine dysautonomia). *Veterinary Record* **134**, 438–440.

Murray, M. J. (1992) Aetiopathogenesis and treatment of peptic ulcer in the horse: a comparative review. *Equine Veterinary Journal* (supplement) **13**, 63–74.

O'Brien, K. (1985) Differential diagnosis of diarrhoea in adult horses. *In Practice* **7**, 53–60.

Proudman, C. J. (1994) The equine tapeworm. *Equine Veterinary Education* **6**, 9–12.

Rumbaugh, G. E., Smith, B. P. & Carlson, G. P. (1978) Internal abdominal abscesses in the horse: a study of 25 cases. *Journal of the American Veterinary Medical Association* **172**, 304–309.

Santschi, E. M., Stone, D. E. Jr & Frank, W. M. (1993) Use of ultrasound in horses for diagnosis of left dorsal displacement of the large colon and monitoring its non surgical correction. *Veterinary Surgery* **22**, 281–284.

Scholes, S. F. E., Vaillant, C., Peacock, P., Edwards, G. B. & Kelly, D. F. (1993) Diagnosis of grass sickness by ileal biopsy. *Veterinary Record* **133**, 7–10.

Siex, M. T. & Wilson, J. H. (1992) Morbidity associated with abdominocentesis – a prospective study. *Equine Veterinary Journal* **13**, 23–25.

White, N. A. (1990) Surgery for acute abdominal disease. In *The Equine Acute Abdomen* (ed. N. A. White) pp. 210–307. Lea & Febiger, Philadelphia.

CHAPTER 7

Diagnosis and Treatment of Sarcoid

DEREK KNOTTENBELT, SUSAN EDWARDS AND
ELIZABETH DANIEL

The term "sarcoid" is derived from the apparent sarcomatous
appearance of the lesions as well as their tendency to recur
following excision. The numbers of sarcoid (previously called
"warts") on any individual animal, their character, distribution
and extent, have a major bearing on the selection of the available treatment options. Clearly, the frustrations felt by many
generations of veterinary surgeons have continued up to the
present time; the equine sarcoid is probably the most common
cutaneous reason for euthanasia and the loss to the equine
industry is considerable. Horses in which there are a few
localized, superficial lesions are usually amenable to any of the
treatment options, although inadequate application will yield a
poor result with a high rate of recurrence at the site and possible
extension to other sites. No effective means of treating the malevolent type of sarcoid has yet been found and interfering with
this particularly aggressive form merely exacerbates the signs.

DIAGNOSIS

A definitive diagnosis of sarcoid can be obtained from biopsy
but the procedure is not without its hazards and in most cases

is not necessary. Sarcoid lesions may be found on all areas of the body but are least common on the dorsum of the trunk.

The equine sarcoid occurs in six distinct forms.

OCCULT SARCOID

The changes due to occult sarcoid lesions are limited to the superficial epidermis with areas (often circular or almost circular) of alopecia with a grey, scaly surface (Fig. 7.1). These are commonly found on the medial thigh, sheath, neck and face but may, like any of the other forms, be found in almost any locality.

Differential diagnosis of occult sarcoid

(1)   Dermatophytosis (ringworm).
(2)   Skin rubs (from tack, stable, etc.).
(3)   Ectoparasites, e.g. lice (lesions are usually pruritic and resolve quickly on treatment).

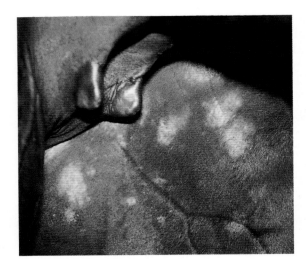

Fig. 7.1 Occult sarcoid on the medial thigh.

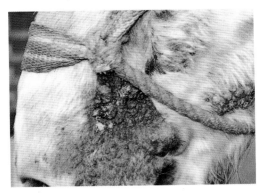

Fig. 7.2 Verrucous sarcoid on the side of the face.

VERRUCOUS SARCOID

An increased epidermal component is evident with verrucous sarcoid, which may be small or very extensive. The lesions are seldom localized, most having an ill-defined margin. The surface has a rough appearance with alternating irregular, thickened, hyperkeratotic areas and flat, scaly areas (Fig. 7.2). The lesions are most often located in the axillae (Fig. 7.3) and groin and occasionally occur elsewhere, such as on the side of the face and at the ear base.

Differential diagnosis of verrucous sarcoid

(1) Equine papillomatosis (grass warts): the difference is sometimes difficult to establish but the course of the two disorders

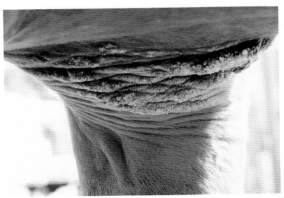

Fig. 7.3 Verrucous sarcoid in the axilla.

is noticeably different – papillomas are self-limiting over 2–3 months at most and are commoner in young horses at grass. Sarcoid persists and continues to expand over a variable period of time.

(2) Hyperkeratosis: from persistent or repeated cutaneous irritation.

(3) Equine sarcoidosis: an exfoliative dermatitis with wasting and generalized, granulomatous inflammation of multiple organ systems similar to the 'lazy leucocyte' syndrome in humans.

(4) Equine molluscum contagiosum: multiple, small, waxy, raised, grey-white, self-limiting papules, which occur primarily in the inguinal and facial regions. Caused by an unclassified poxvirus.

(5) Horsepox: rare, self-limiting, benign disease causing vesicles and crusting around the face, lower limb and genital regions.

(6) Squamous cell carcinoma: cutaneous form.

NODULAR SARCOID

Nodular sarcoid tumours are usually entirely subcutaneous, giving the appearance of spherical (marble-sized, though can be smaller or larger) nodules under intact, apparently normal skin. The overlying skin is often apparently normal but sometimes takes on a thinner, shiny appearance with the mass adherent to the skin (Fig. 7.4). The lesions vary in size, number and

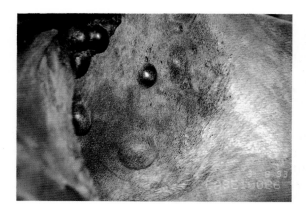

Fig. 7.4 Nodular sarcoid in the groin, some of which is covered by thin, shiny skin.

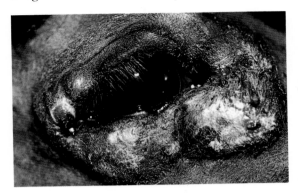

Fig. 7.5 Nodular sarcoid deforming the eyelid margin.

distribution but are most often found in the groin and on the eyelid margins where they may create clinically significant deformities (Fig. 7.5). They may ulcerate, developing quickly into a true fibroblastic sarcoid.

Differential diagnosis of nodular sarcoid

(1) Fibroma.
(2) Neurofibroma: in the upper eyelid, in particular.
(3) Benign dermal or subcutaneous swellings: including hypodermiasis (warble fly) and dermoid cysts.
(4) Allergic (axillary) collagen necrosis: idiopathic, firm intradermal nodules developing in the girth and axillary regions and rarely elsewhere.
(5) Melanoma: usually restricted to grey horses.

FIBROBLASTIC SARCOID

Fibroblastic sarcoid tumours are the most aggressive type, having the appearance of a true neoplasm. The surface is usually ulcerated and is liable to trauma, haemorrhage and local infection (Fig. 7.6). In some cases the extent of the tumour can be easily defined and may have a pedunculated nature (Fig. 7.7). In others, the margins of the tumour are poorly defined and the mass has a sessile and invasive character (Fig. 7.8). The lesions develop at almost any site but in the absence of traumatic skin

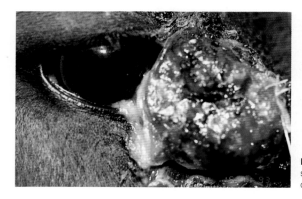

Fig. 7.6 Ulcerated fibroblastic sarcoid associated with conjunctivitis.

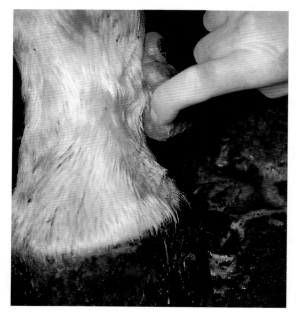

Fig. 7.7 Pedunculated fibroblastic sarcoid on the distal limb.

injuries they are seldom located on the sides of the chest, neck or back. Fibroblastic lesions are relatively common complications of skin wounds, particularly of the limbs (Fig. 7.9). They are also found following accidental or iatrogenic interference (including biopsy) with other forms of sarcoid.

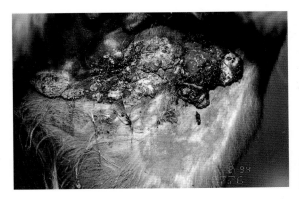

Fig. 7.8 Sessile and locally invasive fibroblastic sarcoid in the axilla.

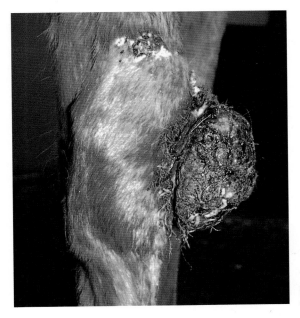

Fig. 7.9 Fibroblastic sarcoid at the site of a previous skin wound.

Differential diagnosis of fibroblastic sarcoid

(1) Exuberant granulation tissue.
(2) Cutaneous botryomycotic lesions: chronic multiple microabscesses due to staphylococcal infection, with exuberant granulation tissue.
(3) Fibrosarcoma.

(4)   Neurofibroma, neurofibrosarcoma.
(5)   Squamous cell carcinoma: palpebral form.

MIXED SARCOID

The mixed form of equine sarcoid consists of an irregular distribution of two or more of the individual types. Mixed sarcoids
are most commonly encountered in the axillae, groin and
around the face (Fig. 7.10).

MALEVOLENT SARCOID

The malevolent form has not previously been described in the
literature as far as the authors are aware. It is a term used to
describe particularly invasive sarcoid tumours which infiltrate
lymphatic vessels resulting in multiple tumour masses along
these vessels and at remote sites such as local lymph nodes.
Usually the malevolent form follows interference with a fibroblastic mass, most often on the elbow or jaw, and rapidly
extends to produce cords of tumour with nodules occurring at
irregular points along their length (Fig. 7.11).

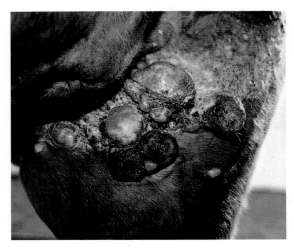

Fig. 7.10 Mixed sarcoid in the
groin made up of fibroblastic,
nodular and occult sarcoid.

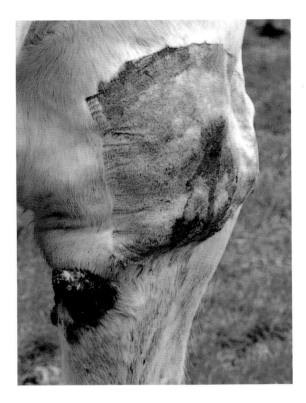

Fig. 7.11 Malevolent form of sarcoid, with multiple cords of tumour tissue extending from a fibroblastic sarcoid on the elbow.

Differential diagnosis of malevolent sarcoid

Lymphangitis: chronic and infectious, including glanders, epizootic lymphangitis and cutaneous histoplasmosis, none of which occur in the UK at present.

PATHOLOGICAL FEATURES

The sarcoid has the capacity for infiltrative expansion in the dermis and subcutis. Histologically, the fibroblastic types have sinuous long pegs of tumour tissue which extend beneath the intact epidermis. Although there are some recognizable differences in the histological appearance between the various forms of sarcoid, the fibroblastic and nodular forms generally resemble fibroma, fibrosarcoma and the rare neurofibroma. Healing of wounds with or without exuberant granulation tissue may be complicated by diffuse or localized sarcoid tissue.

True metastatic spread does not occur, although there are reports of the development of multiple, small lesions following incomplete surgical removal of one or more sarcoid or shortly after the administration of autogenous vaccines. The malevolent form has some characteristics of an aggressive, locally invasive neoplasm.

EPIDEMIOLOGICAL FACTORS

There has been considerable interest in the aetiology of sarcoid and, in particular, the possible role of a virus which is equivocally related to the bovine papillomavirus (BPV) particles. The major problem with this otherwise attractive theory is the failure, thus far, to demonstrate a definitive virus particle in sarcoid lesions. The ability of the BPV to transform fibroblasts in vitro has been demonstrated. Furthermore, the intracutaneous injection of the virus (and, in some cases, cell-free extracts of sarcoid tissue) in horses induces a sarcoid-like lesion; such experimental lesions usually resolve spontaneously and the horse produces detectable antibody to the virus after injection with the virus. In naturally occurring cases neither spontaneous resolution nor antibody to any of the BPV variants has been found. The ability, or otherwise, of the horse to support the vegetative part of the life cycle of the virus may be significant in the pathogenesis of the condition. There is no evidence to suggest that the equine papillomavirus is either related to sarcoid or responsible for the subsequent development of sarcoid. Horses that have had viral papillomata are probably neither more nor less susceptible to the development of sarcoid in later life.

Sarcoid lesions seen in the UK have some noticeable differences from those seen in some other parts of the world. In Australia, for example, it is less common to find horses with large numbers of sarcoid and most studies reported from continental Europe and North America show an average of between two and eight sarcoid lesions per horse. In the UK, it is relatively rare to find horses with single or few lesions; multiple lesions (10 to several thousand) are much more common here than elsewhere. The character of the lesions also appears to have a geographical variation, with occult and verrucous lesions being unusual in Africa, Australia and North America, but particularly common in the UK. The significance of the epidemiological and clinical variations seen in different parts of the world and indeed on different horses in the same geographical locality makes the virus theory on its own somewhat less credible.

There is strong circumstantial evidence that flies are involved in the pathogenesis and epidemiology of the disease, and it is possible that the different biting flies in different geographical areas have some role in the regional variations in numbers and types of sarcoid. They may also have an influence on the spread of sarcoid from horse to horse. In some areas of the world, sarcoid is regarded as a contagious disease.

TREATMENT OPTIONS

Effective therapeutic options for the treatment of sarcoid are very limited and little material progress has been made in either control or treatment. The success of the available treatment options varies between individual veterinary surgeons. In cases where lesions are small and few in number or where they do not interfere with normal function it may be better not to intervene therapeutically. This also applies to cases considered too severe to be treated by any conventional means, but where other factors such as pregnancy, may be a reason for prolonging life.

The methods that are currently available for treatment of the equine sarcoid are outlined below. They have also been reviewed by Marti *et al.* (1993).

SURGICAL REMOVAL

Surgical (sharp) excision is an option favoured by many veterinary surgeons. It has been performed for many years and while some surgeons have had good or excellent results, others have had particularly bad experiences. A major problem associated with surgical treatment is the propensity for regrowth at the site. Furthermore, in some situations, such as with tumours involving the eyelid and distal limb, the option is not usually viable for cosmetic reasons and lack of a suitable means of wound closure or the subsequent interference with normal function (for example, eyelid deformities).

The rate of regrowth of the equine sarcoid following surgical excision is closely dependent upon the extent of the tumour and the degree to which the surgeon can define its limits. Small, well-defined tumours carry the best prognosis for surgical removal, while extensive areas of poorly defined verrucous and mixed sarcoid may result in rapid regrowth of a more aggressive sarcoid type. The worst possible scenario appears to be when single fibroblastic or nodular lesions are removed from a surrounding area of occult or verrucous sarcoid (see Fig. 7.10). The earliest regrowth occurs within days of incomplete excision and is usually accompanied by rapid wound dehiscence and subsequent failure to heal.

While it is not possible to quantify the results generally obtained in practice, most surgeons elect to remove only the most defined lesions in amenable sites and the rate of recurrence under these circumstances is likely to be low. However, cases referred to the University of Liverpool over 5 years have shown that sarcoid regrowth can occur at the site of previous surgery up to 10–15 years later; in over 90% of cases of recurrence, the regrowth was more aggressive in character. There is also a distinct tendency for sarcoid to develop at the site of other skin injuries (see Fig. 7.9), including surgical wounds such as castration incisions.

The surgical excision of nodular sarcoid has, however, been shown to be an effective means of removing single or multiple masses. Regrowth is only likely to occur if the tumour is closely related to the overlying skin and its margins are, therefore, poorly defined or if the mass of the tumour is incised during the procedure; in the case of the latter, regrowth occurs as fibroblastic sarcoid in over 60% of lesions (Fig. 7.12).

Surgical excision of nodular eyelid tumours is not recommended in spite of their apparently benign and circumscribed outward appearance, as they appear to have a particular tendency to develop deep and extensive local infiltration.

The value of carbon dioxide laser excision is uncertain at present and the cosmetic effects, cost and technical dangers are probably still unacceptable.

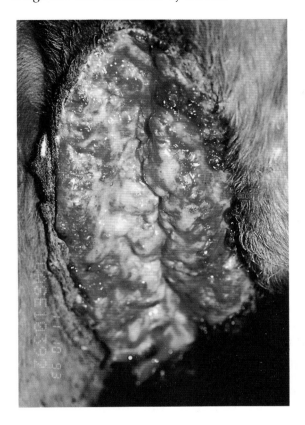

Fig. 7.12 Large mass of ulcerated fibroblastic sarcoid which developed following surgical excision of a nodular sarcoid in the axilla.

CRYOSURGERY

Following cryosurgery, Lane (1977) demonstrated a 44% chance of regrowth. Most surgeons using cryosurgery first surgically debulk larger masses and, again, careful selection of lesions may bias the results heavily in favour of resolution. Extensive areas of superficial sarcoid or large bulky masses of tumour extensively infiltrated into the surrounding skin and subcutis would be unlikely to resolve. Cryosurgery is unsuitable for eyelid tumours or masses overlying joints. The technical complications of accurate cryosurgery, including prolonged general anaesthesia and the need for careful placement of the thermocouples, and the inherent ability of the body to resist freezing, make its practical application less effective than other therapeutic options. When the technique works, the results are usually cosmetically and functionally reasonable, with leucoderma, leucotrichia and some scarring being the only untoward effects.

Crude liquid nitrogen contact cryocautery is commonly resorted to with unpredictable results. In 6% of cases subjected to cryosurgery, Lane (1977) noted a detectable benefit, with complete or partial reduction of sarcoid at remote sites, but this finding has not been commonly encountered and the role of cryoantigens has still to be clarified.

HYPERTHERMIA

Hyperthermia is a rarely reported treatment option and consequently the results are difficult to predict. Tumours require repeated treatments and the benefits are slow to develop. It seems unlikely that this will become a practical means of treatment for any but the smallest lesions and, in any case, this method appears to have no material benefit over any others.

IMMUNE-MEDIATED THERAPY

In theory, immune-mediated therapy (autogenous vaccines and immunomodulation) is a highly attractive option, particularly when one considers a possible viral aetiology. However, autogenous vaccines, which are commonly and effectively used in the treatment of equine viral papillomata, have shown no convincing therapeutic effect. Indeed, there have been suggestions that both the severity and number of lesions may increase dramatically following their use. Autogenous vaccines are not recommended therefore at present.

The use of an immunomodulator, such as BCG cell wall extracts of varying purity, has proved to be a more effective option (Fig. 7.13). The mechanisms involved are unclear and the effects are limited to individually injected tumours. Efficacy is dependent upon an adequate relative volume of antigen being injected directly into the lesion and the response relies upon an effective immune capacity of the host, relatively few tumours and a suitable formulation of the protein. Each tumour has to receive a defined amount of antigen repeatedly; therefore, the technique has limitations of practicality and cost. Usually, successive injections are given at one-, two- and three-week inter-

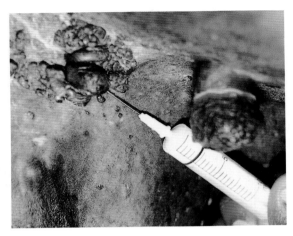

Fig. 7.13 Injection of BCG cell wall extract into a nodular sarcoid.

vals with each subsequent injection being given a further week apart until an effect is observed. A detectable benefit, manifest as swelling and possibly some discharge, is often seen after the second or third dose and further injections may not be necessary. There is an ill-defined, but significant, risk of anaphylaxis following the second or subsequent injections, making prior medication with corticosteroids (e.g. dexamethasone at 0.5 mg/kg intravenously and flunixin meglumine at 1.0 mg/kg intravenously) and close monitoring of the case in the first 12–24 hours after injection, wise precautions. The efficacy is variable with a high reported success rate for periocular tumours but disappointing results elsewhere. There have been suggestions that the use of BCG in the treatment of fibroblastic sarcoid on the lower limb and abdominal wall may exacerbate the tumours.

RADIATION THERAPY

Radiation brachytherapy (using gold 198, radium 226 or iridium 192 sources) has been used for the treatment of equine sarcoid to good effect, particularly in the treatment of periocular sarcoid. At the University of Liverpool over a 5-year period, 45 horses received ^{192}Ir brachytherapy for the treatment of a total of 165 sarcoid lesions in the periorbital area. Four lesions over joints of the lower limb, and one with a lesion in the brisket region which was refractory to several other forms of therapy, were also treated using this method; of these, one case with a palpebral lesion and one with an extensive fibroblastic, sessile sarcoid on the medial aspect of the fore pastern, showed regrowth and required a second treatment. The combined results of the Liverpool studies showed a total resolution of eyelid sarcoid in 49 out of 50 horses (98%) (Fig. 7.14). In the 10 cases with sarcoid tumours at other sites an overall resolution rate of 10 of 11 lesions (91%) was obtained. The efficacy of radiation has been confirmed by other centres, but management and cost implications inevitably restrict its use. The size of the lesion is also a limiting factor as each source can treat only a limited volume of tumour in its immediate vicinity.

The possible application of orthovoltage teletherapy, used for the treatment of other cutaneous neoplasms, and strontium pencil/wand methods has yet to be reported but is probably even more limited by technical requirements and the need to provide repeated doses of radiation which, at present, requires general anaesthesia.

A major advantage of the radiation option is the acceptable cosmetic results with minimal scarring. Apart from some localized alopecia, leucotrichia and leucoderma, the method causes almost no detectable untoward effects.

CHEMOTHERAPY

Topical

The topical application of cytotoxic chemicals for the treatment of equine sarcoid has been widely practised for over a hundred

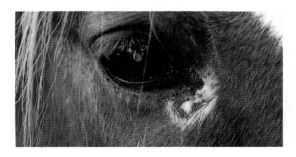

Fig. 7.14 Site of periorbital sarcoid following treatment with iridium 192 brachytherapy. Apart from small areas of alopecia, leucotrichia and leucoderma, the overall cosmetic result is good.

years. A variety of topical cauterizing agents have been used, including sulphuric acid, nitric acid, silver nitrate, mercuric chloride, copper sulphate, arsenic trioxide and several lead and antimony salts and various mixtures of these, podophyllum (a caustic, cytotoxic chemical) and fluorouracil. Trials at the University of Liverpool of a promising topical material have thus far resulted in an overall resolution rate of over 70%. The method relies upon repeated application of a chemical mixture containing a number of heavy metal salts and antimitotic compounds. The mixture is applied in ointment form directly to the surface of sarcoid lesions and results in preferential necrosis and sloughing of the sarcoid tissue over a period of 5–10 weeks. Consistent with other treatment methods, there have been remarkable successes but also significant failures.

Intralesional

Intralesional implants and injections of alkylating agents such as cisplatin are reportedly effective against some types of sarcoid. As with most other topical treatments, the compounds need to be applied at frequent intervals and the results to date have been somewhat disappointing. An intralesional/injectable form of the topical agent being developed at the University of Liverpool has produced some excellent results, particularly in the treatment of nodular and very large fibroblastic sarcoid, with no clinical evidence of systemic toxicity (Fig. 7.15).

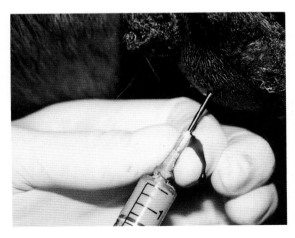

Fig. 7.15 Intralesional injection of cytotoxic cream into a nodular sarcoid.

THE FUTURE

More effective means for the treatment of equine sarcoid are urgently needed. Currently, the efficacy of treatments depends heavily upon the early recognition of sarcoid tumours. Radiation brachytherapy is probably the most effective option, but it is only applicable in a very limited number of cases and under strict control. Conversely, surgical excision, the most widely applied treatment, appears to be the least effective overall. A lack of understanding of the potential severity of the disorder both to the affected horse and to other horses, donkeys and mules with which it comes in contact, often results in lack of treatment. The development of topical agents is only a step forward along a very rocky and perilous path which requires considerable financial input. Any thought of prophylactic measures needs to await the identification of a definitive aetiology.

In the meantime, the term "wart" should not be used when referring to sarcoid skin disease as horse owners are apt to misconstrue the meaning of such a term; "skin cancer" may better convey the severity of the disorder. Prospective purchasers of horses with even limited numbers of sarcoid should be counselled very carefully as to the likely implications.

Acknowledgements

The authors are grateful to colleagues at the University of Liverpool for their continuing assistance and to referring and other interested veterinarians for their support.

REFERENCES AND FURTHER READING

Knottenbelt, D. C. & Pascoe, R. R. (1994) *Colour Atlas of Diseases and Disorders of the Horse*, p. 279. Mosby-Wolfe, London.

Lane, J. G. (1977) The treatment of equine sarcoids by cryosurgery. *Equine Veterinary Journal* **9**, 127–133.

Marti, E., Lazary, S., Antczak, D. F. & Gerber, H. (1993) Report of the first international workshop on equine sarcoid. *Equine Veterinary Journal* **25**, 397–407.

Owen, R. R. & Jagger, D. W. (1987) Clinical observations on the use of BCG cell wall fraction for treatment of periocular and other equine sarcoids. *Veterinary Record* **120**, 548–552.

Wyn-Jones, G. (1979) Treatment of periocular tumours of horses using radioactive gold[196] grains. *Equine Veterinary Journal* **11**, 3–10.

Wyn-Jones, G. (1983) Treatment of equine cutaneous neoplasia by radiotherapy using iridium[192] linear sources. *Equine Veterinary Journal* **15**, 361–365.

CHAPTER 8

Differential Diagnosis of Chronic Coughing

BRUCE McGORUM

Horses with chronic (over 2 months' duration) coughing may present a considerable diagnostic challenge for the equine clinician. As the various causes of chronic coughing necessitate different treatments and have different prognoses, the cause should be determined where possible (Table 8.1). Providing symptomatic treatment alone often gives only temporary clinical improvement.

Table 8.1 Major causes of chronic coughing in the horse.

Chronic obstructive pulmonary disease

Post-infectious airway disease

Lungworm

Pulmonary abscessation and pneumonia

Summer pasture-associated obstructive pulmonary disease (SPAOPD)

Exercise-induced pulmonary haemorrhage

Tracheal collapse

Thoracic neoplasia

CHRONIC OBSTRUCTIVE PULMONARY DISEASE

Chronic obstructive pulmonary disease (COPD), a pulmonary hypersensitivity to inhaled allergens including *Faenia rectivirgula* and *Aspergillus fumigatus*, which are found in poorly saved hay and straw, is by far the most common cause of chronic coughing in horses in the UK. Since the 1980s increased client awareness of COPD and improved air hygiene in stables have resulted in alterations in the manifestations of COPD. Today, affected horses are often presented early in the disease course, when they first exhibit signs of occasional coughing or exercise intolerance. Consequently, fewer cases can be diagnosed confidently from the history and clinical findings alone, resulting in an increased reliance on ancillary diagnostic techniques. The value of clinical examination and ancillary diagnostic techniques is described below.

CLINICAL EXAMINATION

Clinical features of 50 cases of COPD referred to the Royal (Dick) School of Veterinary Studies (R(D)SVS), Edinburgh, in 1990 indicate the diagnostic limitations of clinical examination. Despite all horses with COPD having lower airway inflammation and mucopurulent secretions within the trachea:

only 50% had a nasal discharge, the remainder swallowing their respiratory secretions;
6% inexplicably presented with unilateral nasal discharges;
16% were reported not to cough.

Eight per cent of horses with COPD had neither cough nor nasal discharge, and presented with exercise intolerance or were diagnosed during routine endoscopy.
Only 23% of horses with COPD had an obvious expiratory 'heave' (Fig. 8.1).
Auscultation of the thorax and of the distal cervical trachea, performed during forced breathing (induced by occluding the external nares for 30 seconds), revealed abnormal breath sounds in only 48% and 64% of horses with COPD, respectively.

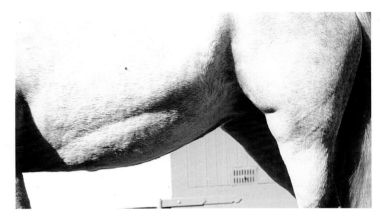

Fig. 8.1 A horse with chronic, severe COPD, showing a 'heave' line. This is a rare finding today, owing to improved recognition and treatment of COPD.

ANCILLARY DIAGNOSTIC TECHNIQUES

BALF analysis

The most valuable diagnostic feature of COPD is a marked neutrophilia of bronchoalveolar lavage fluid (BALF) (i.e. > 5% neutrophils) and of tracheal aspirates (commonly > 90% neutrophils). These analyses are readily performed in equine practice. While tracheal aspirates are easier to collect than BALF, BALF cytology is easier to interpret and usually provides more diagnostically useful information (Table 8.2).

To aid detection of mild COPD, clinical and BALF cytological examinations may be performed 24 hours after housing horses in a stable containing mouldy hay and straw. After this challenge, horses with COPD show a marked BALF neutrophilia and usually an exacerbation of clinical symptoms.

Endoscopy

While endoscopy always reveals accumulations of mucopurulent secretions within the distal trachea of horses with COPD, this is a feature of most equine pulmonary diseases and is not pathognomonic for COPD (Fig. 8.2).

Table 8.2 Bronchoalveolar lavage fluid (BALF) and tracheal aspirate cytological findings in horses with chronic pulmonary disease.

Normal cytology:
  Normal horse
  Chronic post-infectious airway disease (however, a transient – i.e. for up to 2 weeks after infection – neutrophilia of BALF and tracheal aspirates is often observed in acute post-infectious airway disease)

Neutrophilia (i.e. > 5% neutrophils in BALF or > 60% in tracheal aspirate):
  COPD
  SPAOPD
  Bacterial bronchopneumonia (intracellular bacteria and toxic neutrophils may be identified)

Eosinophilia (i.e. > 3% eosinophils):
  Lungworm
  Idiopathic pulmonary eosinophilia (rare)

Haemosiderophages:
  EIPH

COPD, chronic obstructive pulmonary disease; SPAOPD, summer pasture-associated obstructive pulmonary disease; EIPH, exercise-induced pulmonary haemorrhage.

Blood gas analysis

While horses with severe COPD show hypoxaemia ($Pao_2 < 85$ mmHg), this finding is not pathognomonic for COPD. Arterial blood gas analysis is rarely performed in equine practice, owing to the expense of equipment and technical problems.

Intrathoracic pressure measurement

The degree of dyspnoea shown by horses with COPD may be quantified in the field by recording intrathoracic pressure changes (Ventigraph, Boehringer Ingelheim). While this is a more valuable technique for assessing dyspnoea than visual examination (Fig. 8.3), at the R(D)SVS only 50% of horses with COPD have shown elevations above the critical level of 6 mmHg reported by McPherson *et al.* (1978). Furthermore, as increased intrathoracic pressure changes have also occasionally been found in horses with other severe lung diseases, this finding is not pathognomonic for COPD.

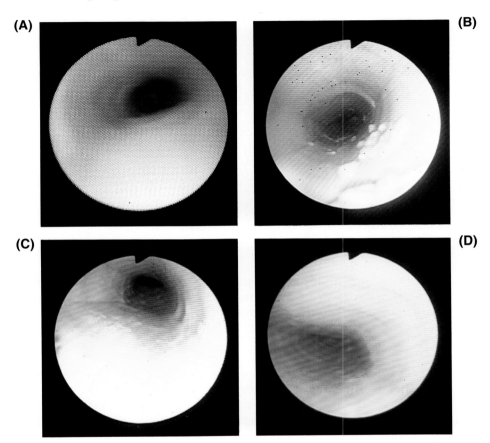

Fig. 8.2 Endoscopic appearance of the trachea of four horses exhibiting chronic coughing. (A) Mucopurulent secretions in a horse with COPD. The presence of mucopurulent secretions indicates that this horse has pulmonary disease, but does not indicate the nature of the disease; grossly similar secretions may be observed in horses with post-infectious airway disease, lungworm and SPAOPD. (B) Tenacious mucopurulent secretions, suggestive of bacterial bronchopneumonia. (C) Lungworms within tracheal lavage fluid in a horse with *Dictyocaulus arnfieldi* infection. Ivermectin had been administered to the horse 3 days previously. (D) Dorsoventral tracheal collapse in an aged pony. Mucopurulent secretions within the distal trachea indicate that this pony has concomitant pulmonary disease.

Immunological methods

Some commercial laboratories can quantify IgE antibodies to mould allergens in equine serum and BALF, but this is of limited diagnostic value because there is overlap in the levels of these antibodies in normal and COPD-affected horses.

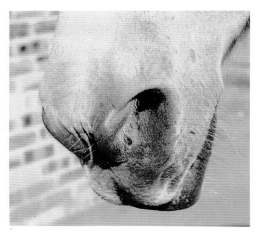

Fig. 8.3 The dilated nostrils of a dyspnoeic horse.

Intradermal mould antigen testing is not of value in the diagnosis of COPD. Many normal horses show positive intradermal reactions to mould antigens and there is limited correlation between the dermal and pulmonary reactivities to mould antigens.

Other techniques

Diagnostic techniques commonly performed in the investigation of chronic coughing, but which rarely yield valuable information, include routine haematology, bacterial culture of nasal swabs and bacterial culture of BALF.

MANAGEMENT OF COPD

Given adequate and permanent exclusion from the causal mould allergens, virtually all horses with COPD can achieve a complete and permanent remission from clinical and laboratory evidence of pulmonary disease. One unfortunate consequence of this is that adequately controlled COPD cannot be detected during pre-purchase examinations and clinical disease may only become evident when the horse is subsequently exposed to allergens.

Unfortunately, chemotherapy is widely overused in the control of COPD. It should be stressed that while bronchodilators may be of value in horses with severe COPD, they are only adjuncts to environmental control. There is no indication for antibiotic therapy in the control of COPD. While it has been reported that hyposensitization with mould allergens may have a beneficial effect on COPD, there has been no adequately controlled study to evaluate this therapy.

Important factors in the control of COPD

All potential sources of the causal mould allergens must be eliminated. This is most easily achieved by keeping horses permanently at pasture. If this is not possible, the bedding, feed, ventilation and surrounding environment must *all* be considered (Fig. 8.4).

Bedding

Shavings or paper bedding should be used and all wet bedding removed daily. Deep litter shavings or paper must be avoided as they rapidly develop heavy mould contamination.

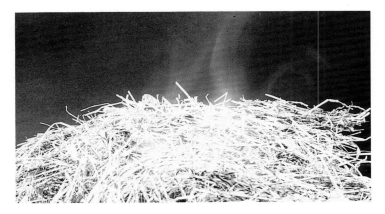

Fig. 8.4 Mould spores liberated from poorly saved hay and straw are the major cause of equine COPD.

Feed

Haylage (high dry matter silage), chopped dried alfalfa, silage
or complete cubed diets are suitable feedstuffs. Feeding soaked
hay is ineffective as the spore challenge is not fully eliminated
and, additionally, the nutritive content of the hay is reduced.

Ventilation

The top door of the stable should be kept open at all times and
there should be a louvred vent (at least 0.3 m²) in the back wall.

Surrounding environment

Affected horses should be kept as far as possible from potential
sources of allergens including stables containing hay and straw,
and dungheaps and barns.

POST-INFECTIOUS AIRWAY DISEASE

Chronic airway disease may be a sequel to infections with respiratory viruses or mycoplasmas. Some clinicians use the term
"inflammatory airway disease" to describe this condition. While
most horses show a remission of clinical symptoms within a
couple of weeks after viral infection, some horses continue
coughing for several months. This chronic coughing may reflect
viral damage to the airway epithelium, which can take several
weeks or months to resolve. Alternatively, it may be due to
virus-induced non-specific bronchial hyperreactivity, which
manifests as coughing and exaggerated bronchospasm in
response to exercise and to inhaled agents including dust, cold
air and dry air.

Affected horses usually have a history of a preceding viral
respiratory disease of acute onset (coughing, nasal discharge,
pyrexia, enlarged submandibular lymph nodes), often with several horses in a group affected. However, this history is not
pathognomonic for this condition as horses that develop COPD
or pulmonary abscessation following viral infections may also

present with similar histories. Diagnosis of chronic post-infectious airway disease may be confirmed by demonstrating a recent seroconversion to a respiratory virus and a normal differential cytology (i.e. absence of neutrophilia) in tracheal mucus and BALF. Culture of viruses from the respiratory tract of horses with chronic post-infectious airway disease is unsuccessful because viruses are usually excreted for only 24–72 hours after infection.

The treatment of post-infectious airway disease includes rest and provision of a dust-free environment. The latter will reduce non-specific bronchial hyperreactivity to inhaled dust and may prevent the subsequent development of COPD, which has been reported as a sequel to viral infections. Some horses with chronic post-infectious airway disease respond favourably to treatment with oral prednisolone (1 mg/kg for 3 weeks, then tail off over a 2-week period). It would be prudent to rule out primary bacterial infection (see below) prior to commencing prednisolone therapy.

LUNGWORM

Lungworm infection is an uncommon condition, usually seen in the late summer or autumn in horses pastured with donkeys, which are the natural, and usually asymptomatic, reservoir hosts of *Dictyocaulus arnfieldi*. Infections in horses are usually non-patent and, consequently, the Baermann faecal flotation technique is unreliable. Diagnosis may be confirmed by demonstrating an eosinophilia (> 3%) in tracheal mucus or BALF, by endoscopic visualization of larvae within the trachea or in collected respiratory secretions (see Fig. 8.2C), or by the response to anthelmintic therapy. Affected horses, and in-contact horses and donkeys, should be given a single dose of ivermectin (Eqvalan, MSD Agvet) at 200 µg/kg, and moved to clean pasture.

BACTERIAL INFECTIONS OF THE EQUINE RESPIRATORY TRACT

LOW-GRADE BACTERIAL INFLAMMATION OF THE LOWER AIRWAYS

Streptococcus zooepidemicus, *Pasteurella/Actinobacillus*-like species and *Streptococcus pneumoniae* appear to be common causes of lower airway inflammation, mild coughing and loss of performance in young racehorses in the UK (Burrell and MacKintosh, 1986; Woods *et al.*, 1993). This area warrants further investigation. *Streptococcus zooepidemicus* may also cause primary chronic pneumonia in older horses. This may be confirmed by culturing a relatively pure growth of this organism from aseptically collected tracheal secretions. Affected horses should be treated with a prolonged (> 10 days) course of penicillin.

PULMONARY ABSCESSATION AND BACTERIAL PNEUMONIA

Pulmonary abscessation and severe bacterial pneumonia of adult horses are rare in the UK in comparison with the USA. Most commonly, these are sequelae to other diseases, especially conditions which cause aspiration of food or saliva (e.g. oesophageal choke), although some primary cases follow strenuous exercise or long-distance travel which impair pulmonary defence mechanisms.

Horses with pulmonary abscessation and severe pneumonia present with a variety of symptoms including dyspnoea, pyrexia, inappetence, lethargy, coughing, thoracic pain, submandibular lymphadenopathy and purulent nasal discharge. Secondary pleuritis may occur in some cases.

Lower respiratory tract bacterial infections are diagnosed by demonstrating significant numbers of bacteria in tracheal mucus following aerobic and anaerobic culture. Ideally, to avoid contamination with nasopharyngeal bacteria, tracheal secretions for bacteriological analysis should be collected aseptically by transtracheal puncture. However, careful endoscopic collection of tracheal aspirates using a sterile endoscope and catheter is a satisfactory practical alternative and carries less risk of complications.

Horses with pulmonary abscessation and pneumonia may be further evaluated using thoracic radiography (rarely feasible except in referral centres); ultrasonography (normal aerated lung does not conduct ultrasound and, therefore, only lesions that are in contact with visceral pleura may be imaged) (Fig. 8.5); endoscopy (purulent discharge may be identified in the trachea or even emanating from the affected lung segment) (see Fig. 8.2B) and haematology (leucocytosis or leucopenia,

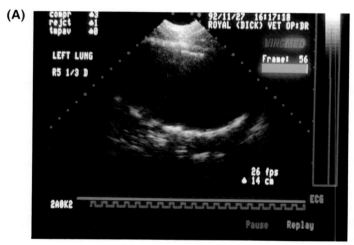

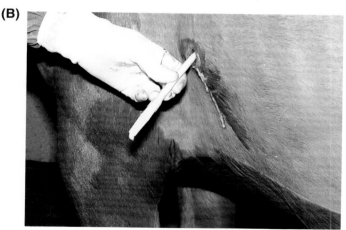

Fig. 8.5 (A) Ultrasonogram of the cranioventral region of the caudal lobe of the left lung. The lung is adherent to the parietal pleura and contains a large abscess, which appears as a hypoechoic mass containing echogenic debris, surrounded by a hyperechoic capsule. (B) Percutaneous drainage of the abscess yielded 4 litres of pus. Culture of this material yielded *Streptococcus zooepidemicus*.

hyperfibrinogenaemia, hyperglobulinaemia, hypoalbuminaemia and mild anaemia are common non-specific findings).

Pulmonary abscessation and severe bacterial pneumonia are
associated with a high mortality rate, necessitating early diagnosis and aggressive treatment. Antibiotic therapy should be
selected on the basis of culture results. Prior to receiving the
culture results, initial antibiotic therapy may be instigated based
on the results of a Gram-stained smear of tracheal secretions.
Alternatively, suitable choices for initial antimicrobial therapy
are potentiated sulphonamides, or, when aspiration and anaerobic bacteria are suspected, penicillin and metronidazole. Affected horses should be fully rested.

SUMMER PASTURE-ASSOCIATED OBSTRUCTIVE PULMONARY DISEASE

Summer pasture-associated obstructive pulmonary disease
(SPAOPD) is an enigmatic condition with similar clinicopathological findings to COPD, but affects pastured horses with no
access to hay and straw. An important feature of SPAOPD is its
seasonality; most horses are affected between spring and early
autumn and show complete or marked remission during winter
months, although many are affected in subsequent years. While
affected horses may present with chronic coughing, severe
dyspnoea is the predominant clinical feature. Crackles and
wheezes are commonly detected on thoracic and tracheal auscultation (Fig. 8.6). Diagnosis can usually be made on the basis
of history and clinical findings, although the marked neutrophilia of tracheal mucus and BALF may be helpful.

Although the aetiology of SPAOPD is unknown, a pulmonary
hypersensitivity to inhaled pollens or outdoor moulds is suspected because SPAOPD and COPD have similar clinicopathological features. Intradermal antigen testing with a wide variety
of antigens has, however, failed to identify the cause. In this
respect, while exposure to oilseed rape (*Brassica* species) antigens can exacerbate pulmonary disease in horses with underlying pulmonary inflammation, this agent does not appear to be
a significant primary cause of equine pulmonary disease
(McGorum and Dixon, 1992).

Currently, the treatment of SPAOPD is unrewarding. Often
the most effective treatment is to move the horse to a different

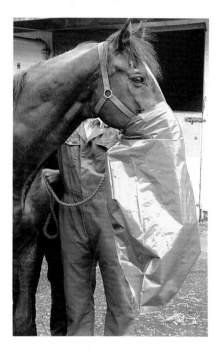

Fig. 8.6 Auscultation of the equine lung field is a relatively insensitive technique since a considerable proportion of the breath sounds are reflected and attenuated by the thick chest wall. The audibility of breath sounds, and hence the sensitivity of auscultation, may be increased by performing auscultation either while the horse is breathing into a rebreathing bag or while it is hyperventilating following a period of nasal occlusion. Additionally, coughing or excessive hyperventilation noted during these procedures are indicative of respiratory disease. Auscultation over the distal cervical trachea can also provide much useful information, since there is only minor attenuation of breath sounds at this site.

environment. If this is not feasible, the horse should be housed in a dust-free environment. Long-acting parenteral cortico-steroids or alternate day oral prednisolone therapy can be very beneficial, although because of their potential side-effects (especially the induction of laminitis) they should be used with caution. Bronchodilators may be of value in dyspnoeic animals, but commonly give only a partial and temporary improvement.

EXERCISE-INDUCED PULMONARY HAEMORRHAGE

While the main presenting signs of exercise-induced pulmonary haemorrhage (EIPH) are pulmonary haemorrhage, occasional epistaxis and, possibly, loss of performance, some affected horses also show chronic coughing. This may reflect concomitant small airway disease, although whether this is a cause of or a sequel to EIPH is not known. In older horses, coughing may indicate underlying COPD.

TRACHEAL COLLAPSE

Tracheal collapse most commonly affects small ponies, especially Shetlands, over 10 years old. Clinical signs include chronic coughing, inspiratory stridor, 'honking' inspiratory and expiratory noise, dyspnoea and cyanosis. These symptoms are often exaggerated during warm weather and by exercise.

Diagnosis of the dorsoventral tracheal flattening may be made by palpation, endoscopy (see Fig. 8.2D), radiography or fluoroscopy, although intermittent dynamic collapse may be more difficult to confirm. As both the cervical and thoracic segments of the trachea are usually involved, treatment such as tracheal imbrication, extraluminal support and tracheal prostheses is generally unsuccessful. Exercise of affected animals should be restricted, expecially in warm weather.

THORACIC NEOPLASIA

Thoracic neoplasia is rare in horses (Fig. 8.7). Most cases involve lymphosarcoma or metastatic disease, with primary lung neoplasia being extremely uncommon. Clinical signs are variable and include weight loss, anorexia, pyrexia, dyspnoea, chronic coughing, pleural effusion, ventral oedema and jugular disten-

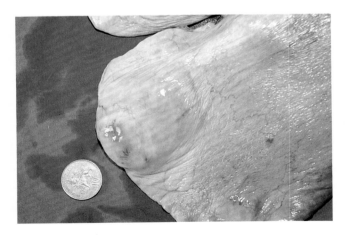

Fig. 8.7 Metastatic squamous cell carcinoma in the caudal left lung; the primary neoplasm affected the penis. This horse showed no clinical signs of pulmonary disease.

sion. Thoracic radiography, ultrasonography, thoracocentesis, pleuroscopy and cytology of pleural fluid or a tracheobronchial aspirate may be of diagnostic value.

MISCELLANEOUS PULMONARY DISEASES

Rare causes of chronic equine coughing include foreign bodies, eosinophilic interstitial pneumonia, pulmonary hydatidosis and pulmonary infarction.

Acknowledgements

Dr P. M. Dixon, Dr E. M. Milne and Mr D. I. Railton are gratefully acknowledged for their helpful comments.

REFERENCES

Burrell, M. H. & MacKintosh, M. E. (1986) Isolation of *Streptococcus pneumoniae* from the respiratory tract of horses. *Equine Veterinary Journal* **18**, 183–186.

McGorum, B. C. & Dixon, P. M. (1992) Preliminary observations on inhalation and intradermal challenges of horses with oil seed rape. *Veterinary Record* **131**, 163–167.

McPherson, E. A., Lawson, G. H. K., Murphy, J. R., Nicholson, J., Breeze, R. G. & Pirie, H. M. (1978) Chronic obstructive pulmonary disease (COPD): identification of affected horses. *Equine Veterinary Journal* **10**, 47–53.

Woods, J. L. N., Burrell, M. H., Roberts, C. A., Chanter, N. & Shaw, Y. (1993) Streptococci and *Pasteurella* species associated with disease of the equine lower respiratory tract. *Equine Veterinary Journal* **25**, 314–318.

CHAPTER 9

Differential Diagnosis and Treatment of Acute Onset Coughing

TIM MAIR

Diseases of the respiratory tract are some of the commonest diseases encountered in horses, and constitute a frequent cause of wastage and time off work. The horse affected by respiratory disease may demonstrate a number of clinical signs including coughing, nasal discharge, laboured breathing, adventitious noise and exercise intolerance. Of these, the cough is the sign most commonly noticed by owners, and the sign most consistently recognized in contagious and lower respiratory tract diseases.

This chapter describes the differential diagnosis and treatment of acute onset coughing in adult horses. Many of the diseases that result in chronic coughing may, potentially, have an acute onset; these are described in Chapter 8. The major causes of acute onset coughing in the older foal and adult horse are listed in Table 9.1.

DIAGNOSTIC APPROACH TO ACUTE ONSET COUGHING

HISTORY

An accurate history can provide valuable clues to the cause of sudden onset coughing (Table 9.2). Many of the diseases have

Table 9.1 Causes of acute onset coughing in older foals and adult horses.

Common	Uncommon (or exotic)

Viral infections:
    equine herpesvirus 1 and 4
    equine influenza
	Adenovirus
	Rhinovirus
	(Equine viral arteritis)
	(African horse sickness)

Strangles (*Streptococcus equi*)	
Bacterial lower respiratory tract infection	Lungworm
Choke, dysphagia	Exercise-induced pulmonary haemorrhage

Acute airway obstruction:
    chronic obstructive pulmonary
        disease
    summer pasture-associated
        obstructive pulmonary disease
	Pleuropneumonia, pneumonia,
	    pulmonary abscess, *Rhodococcus*
	    equi pneumonia
	Inhaled foreign bodies

Acute pharyngitis, laryngitis	Tracheal collapse, constriction
	Rupture of mitral chordae tendineae
	Pulmonary oedema

a marked age prevalence. *Rhodococcus equi*, for example, causes pneumonia in the older foal (up to 6 months of age); this infection also tends to be endemic on certain farms, so a history of previous problems on the premises can be helpful. Clinical equine herpesvirus (EHV) infections and strangles are commonest in weanlings, yearlings and young adults, while acute airway obstruction associated with chronic obstructive pulmonary disease (COPD) or summer pasture-associated obstructive pulmonary disease (SPAOPD) is most likely to affect mature horses.

A history of recent contact with other horses at shows, sales, etc., might indicate an infectious condition; stress due to transportation, surgery, etc., can also predispose horses to infectious diseases, including pneumonia and pleuropneumonia. Environmental conditions may be relevant (Fig. 9.1). Acute airway obstruction associated with COPD occurs in stabled horses, whereas SPAOPD and lungworm are diseases of pastured horses. A history of recent or current shared grazing with donkeys is usual in lungworm cases. The season and weather conditions can also be helpful. Clinical signs of COPD are usually seen in the autumn and winter, and acute exacerbations are

Table 9.2 History: factors that may aid diagnosis.

	EHV infection	Influenza	Strangles	BLRTI	COPD	SPAOPD	Lungworm	Adult pneumonia	R. equi pneumonia
Age									
Less than 6 months	+	+	+	+			+		+++
Young adults	+++	+++	+++	+++	+++	+	+++	+++	
Mature	+	++	+	+	+++	+++	+++	+++	
Contagious spread	++	+++	+++	++			+		+
Environment									
Stable					+++				
Pasture						+++	+++		
Donkey contact							+++		
Previous disease									++
Stress	+	+	++					+++	
Season									
Summer/autumn					++	+++	+++		++
Autumn/winter					+++				

Key: +, sometimes; ++, commonly; +++, very commonly; EHV, equine herpesvirus; BLRTI, bacterial lower respiratory tract infection; COPD, chronic obstructive pulmonary disease; SPAOPD, summer pasture-associated obstructive pulmonary disease; R. equi, Rhodococcus equi.

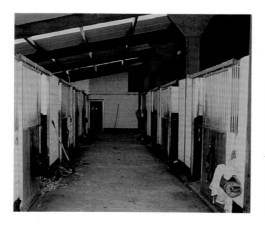

Fig. 9.1 The housing of large numbers of horses in close proximity to each other and in a shared airspace aids the spread of contagious diseases among susceptible animals. The difficulties in achieving adequate ventilation rates in barn systems as shown here result in high concentrations of airborne environmental contaminants and allergens, which are further detrimental to respiratory health. Coughing and respiratory diseases tend to be common in horses housed under these conditions.

frequently associated with sudden changes in weather conditions. Lungworm infection and SPAOPD are usually seen in the summer and autumn.

CLINICAL FEATURES

The nature of the cough and other clinical signs may be helpful in reaching a diagnosis (Table 9.3). Harsh, dry or hacking coughs usually originate from upper respiratory tract infections (especially viral infections), whereas soft, deep and productive coughs usually originate from the lower respiratory tract. Swallowing after coughing is indicative of a productive cough. Coughing while eating suggests pharyngeal or laryngeal inflammation (which might be secondary to lower respiratory tract disease), or aspiration of food. Painful, short coughs can be observed in viral infections and pleuritis.

If present, the nature of the nasal discharge should be noted. Serous discharges are typical of early viral infections, but they commonly become mucopurulent later owing to secondary bacterial infection (Fig. 9.2). Mucopurulent discharges are also seen in many lower respiratory tract diseases. Purulent discharges occur in horses with strangles and bronchopneumonia or lung abscesses. A malodorous discharge suggests guttural pouch infection, pneumonia, lung abscess or an inhaled foreign body. The presence of food material in the discharge indicates dysphagia (e.g. choke, strangles or guttural pouch mycosis).

Table 9.3 Clinical features that may aid diagnosis.

	Viral infection	Strangles	BLRTI	Acute airway obstruction	Choke	Acute pharyngitis	Lung-worm	EIPH	Adult pneumonia	R. equi pneumonia	Foreign body	Tracheal collapse
Cough												
Dry	+++		+++	+++		+++				+	+	+++
Productive	+	++	+++	+	+++		++	+	++	++	++	
Painful	+	+			+	+			+++			
Inappetence	++	++	+		+++	+			+++	++		
Weight loss	+	+			+				++	++		
Nasal discharge												
Serous	+++	+				+						
Mucopurulent	++	+++	++	+		+	++		+++	+	++	
Purulent		+++			+++				++	+	++	
Food		+			+++							
Malodour					+				++		+++	
Blood								+++	+		+	
Dyspnoea												
Inspiratory		++			+	+			+++	+++	+	+++
Expiratory		+	+	+++			+		+++	+++	+	
Stridor		++				+					+	+++

Key: +, sometimes; ++, commonly; +++, very commonly; BLRTI, bacterial lower respiratory tract infection; EIPH, exercise-induced pulmonary haemorrhage; R. equi, Rhodococcus equi.

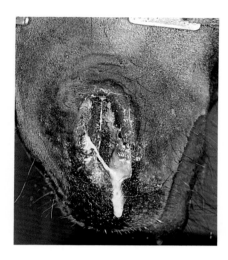

Fig. 9.2 Mucopurulent nasal discharge typical of bacterial infection in a horse with viral upper respiratory tract disease.

The presence or absence of dyspnoea and, if present, its nature, are important observations. Sudden onset coughing without dyspnoea is typical of upper respiratory tract infections (in particular viral infections). Coughing with inspiratory dyspnoea is seen in upper airway obstructions such as pharyngeal paralysis, laryngeal or tracheal trauma, and tracheal collapse, whereas coughing with expiratory dyspnoea is typical of lower (acute) airway obstruction. A cough with both inspiratory and expiratory dyspnoea indicates concurrent upper and lower airway disease, or overwhelming thoracic disease such as pleuropneumonia.

Clinical examination

A full clinical examination is necessary to determine the presence of systemic signs and evidence of disease in other body systems (Table 9.4). Pyrexia occurs in many infectious diseases, but is a variable feature of pneumonia. Submandibular lymph node enlargement is also common in infectious diseases, but can be an indication of neoplastic infiltration. Abscessation of the glands may occur in strangles or some secondary bacterial infections.

The laryngeal cough reflex shows increased sensitivity in many infective or inflammatory airway diseases. Auscultation

Table 9.4 Findings of the clinical examination that may aid diagnosis.

	Viral infection	Strangles	BLRTI	Acute airway obstruction	Choke	Acute pharyngitis	Lung-worm	EIPH	Pneu-monias	Foreign body	Tracheal collapse	Ruptured chordae tendineae
Pyrexia	+++	+++	++						++			
Submandibular lymph nodes												
Enlargement	+++	+++	++			+			+			
Abscesses	+	+++										
Laryngeal cough reflex	+++	+++	+++	+++	++	+++	+		++	+	+	
Lung sounds												
Harshness	+	+	++	+++			++	+	+++	++	++	++
Crackles			+	+++			+	+	+++		+++	+++
Wheezes			+	+++			+		+++			
Ventral dullness									++			
Heart murmur												+++
Chest percussion												
Pain									+++	+		
Ventral dullness									+++			

Key: +, sometimes; ++, commonly; +++, very commonly; BLRTI, bacterial lower respiratory tract infection; EIPH, exercise-induced pulmonary haemorrhage.

of the chest should be performed in a quiet environment, and the entire lung fields as well as the heart should be auscultated on both sides of the chest. Adventitious lung sounds include crackles and wheezes, which indicate small airway obstruction; they may be heard in many lung diseases including acute airway obstruction and pneumonia. An absence of lung sounds in the ventral chest is suggestive of pleural effusion. Sudden onset coughing associated with a loud pansystolic heart murmur (and sometimes arrhythmia due to atrial fibrillation) might indicate ruptured mitral chordae tendineae. Percussion of the chest is limited in the adult horse, but a pain response is often observed in early pleuritis, and ventral dullness suggests pleural effusion.

FURTHER DIAGNOSTIC TESTS

Further tests that can aid diagnosis include the following:

 (1)   Haematology.
 (2)   Bacterial culture.
 (3)   Virus isolation.
 (4)   Virus serology.
 (5)   Demonstration of viral antigens.
 (6)   Endoscopy.
 (7)   Tracheal aspiration.
 (8)   Bronchoalveolar lavage.
 (9)   Radiography.
(10)   Ultrasonography.

Routine haematology often reveals non-specific changes in the white cells in infectious diseases. A leucopenia with a reversal of the neutrophil–lymphocyte ratio and monocytosis are suggestive of viral infections, whereas a leucocytosis with neutrophilia is indicative of bacterial infections.

Bacterial cultures of transtracheal aspirates are helpful in lower respiratory tract infections, and should always be performed in cases of pneumonia. Cultures from lymph node abscesses yield *Streptococcus equi* in strangles. Bacterial cultures of nasal swabs are rarely helpful unless a specific pathogen is identified; *S. equi* may be isolated from this site in strangles cases, but the organism is frequently swamped by other bacteria, and its isolation from an abscess may be more reliable.

Endoscopy is helpful in the diagnosis of many diseases including pharyngitis and laryngitis, inhaled foreign bodies, guttural pouch disease, pharyngeal paralysis, tracheal collapse, lungworm and lower airway infection. Tracheal aspiration and bronchoalveolar lavage are useful tests for the diagnosis of lower airway infection, lungworm, COPD and SPAOPD (see Chapter 8).

DIFFERENTIAL DIAGNOSIS OF ACUTE ONSET COUGHING

VIRAL INFECTIONS

Most horses that suddenly start coughing are affected by an upper respiratory tract viral infection. The most important viral infections in the UK are EHV and equine influenza. Equine viral arteritis (EVA) appears to be endemic at a low level among standardbred horses in the UK, but recent outbreaks in other breeds have been recognized and its reintroduction in the future is possible. African horse sickness is exotic to the UK, but recent outbreaks in Europe and the Middle East give cause for concern that it could spread. The clinical features of these viral infections are summarized in Table 9.5.

Equine rhinopneumonitis (EHV)

Equine herpesviruses 1 and 4 (formerly classified as subtypes 1 and 2 of EHV-1) are constantly circulating within the horse population. These viruses are capable of establishing latent infections, which may be reactivated by stress. Furthermore, immunity following infection is short-lived, and horses may be reinfected many times throughout their lives. Clinical respiratory disease is most marked in young horses; in older horses, infection may be subclinical or associated with exercise intolerance. Infection with EHV-1 can result in abortion (sometimes causing "abortion storms"), neonatal illness and neurological disease, in addition to respiratory disease. Infection with EHV-4 is most commonly associated with respiratory disease, although sporadic cases of abortion have been reported.

Table 9.5 Clinical features of important respiratory viral infections.

Viral infection	Clinical features	Specific diagnosis
Adenovirus	Subclinical in adults. May cause severe respiratory disease (cough, nasal discharge, pyrexia, diarrhoea) in foals. Common cause of pneumonia in Arabian foals with combined immunodeficiency	Virus isolation (nasopharyngeal and conjunctival swabs) Viral antigens in nasal and conjunctival smears Intranuclear inclusions in smears (nasal/conjunctival) Serology
EHV-1 and 4	Significant contagious respiratory disease in weanlings and yearlings – pyrexia (up to 40.5 °C/105 °F), serous nasal discharge, becoming mucopurulent, cough. Less severe or subclinical disease in older horses. Viral pneumonia in newborns. Also associated with abortion and neurological disease (EHV-1)	Virus isolation (nasopharyngeal swabs, plasma) Serology Histology of fetal tissues (intranuclear inclusions) Immunofluorescence/immunoperoxidase to detect viral antigens in tissues
Equine influenza	Rapid spread among susceptible horses. Pyrexia (up to 41 °C/106 °F), anorexia, lethargy, harsh dry cough, serous nasal discharge becoming mucopurulent. Less severe or subclinical disease in vaccinated horses	Virus isolation (nasopharyngeal swabs) Serology Detection of viral antigens in nasal swabs, nasal washings and tracheal aspirates (e.g. ELISA test)

Rhinovirus	Mild clinical or subclinical respiratory disease. May be identified in association with other viral infections	Virus isolation (nasopharyngeal swabs) Serology
Equine viral arteritis	Variable signs; may be subclinical. Pyrexia (up to 41 °C/106 °F), oedema (especially periorbital, limbs and scrotum), ocular and nasal discharges, anorexia, skin rash, cough, diarrhoea, abortion. Carrier state in stallions	Virus isolation (nasopharyngeal and conjunctival swabs, buffy coat cells, fetal tissues, semen) Serology
African horse sickness	Peracute (pulmonary form): pyrexia, respiratory distress, cough, frothy nasal discharge, rapidly fatal Subacute (cardiac form): pyrexia, periorbital, neck and thoracic oedema Petechial haemorrhages	Virus isolation (heparinized blood or tissue) ELISA to demonstrate viral antigens in tissues Serology

EHV, equine herpesvirus; ELISA, enzyme-linked immunosorbent assays.

Equine influenza

The widespread use of killed vaccines has significantly reduced the extent and severity of equine influenza. However, as a result of the constant movement and mixing of horses within and between countries, influenza remains a persistent risk. Two antigenically distinct subtypes of the virus exist, A/equine/1 (H7N7) and A/equine/2 (H3N8). Continued antigenic drift of the A/equine/2 (H3N8) virus subtype is one reason for the recurrence of epizootics of influenza. The last major outbreak in the UK, in 1989, was due to an antigenically drifted variant, which resulted in infection in both vaccinated and unvaccinated horses. Influenza is currently endemic in the UK, but at a low level. Outbreaks are most common during the summer when large numbers of horses mix at shows and events.

Infection of vaccinated horses can result in virus shedding in the absence of clinical signs, and this may be an important source of infection for other susceptible horses. Outbreaks among susceptible or unvaccinated horses can be explosive, reflecting the release and aerosolization of vast amounts of virus by frequent coughing, and the short (1–3 days) incubation period.

Equine viral arteritis

The clinical features of equine arteritis virus infection are highly variable and in areas where the virus is endemic subclinical infection is common. Clinical signs of EVA include pyrexia, depression, anorexia, conjunctivitis ("pinkeye") and lacrimation (Fig. 9.3), serous nasal discharge, coughing, ataxia, diarrhoea, skin rash and oedema of the limbs, ventral abdomen, scrotum/mammary gland and periorbital areas. Pregnant mares (3–10 months of gestation) may abort at the time of, or shortly after, infection, and abortion storms can occur.

Equine arteritis virus is generally transmitted by the respiratory route, although infected stallions may become carriers, shedding the organism in their semen and resulting in venereal infection of mares after natural mating or artificial insemination. Approximately 30% of seropositive stallions become carriers, and this state can persist for years after the initial infection.

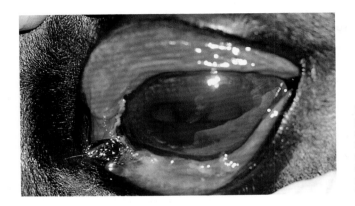

Fig. 9.3 Conjunctivitis ("pinkeye") with excessive lacrimation is commonly seen in equine viral arteritis, although the clinical presentation is highly variable.

Diagnosis of viral infections

The diagnosis of viral infections is usually presumptive, based on the history and clinical signs. A specific diagnosis is often not required since there is no therapeutic benefit to be gained from knowing which virus is involved; furthermore, the results of laboratory tests may take several weeks, by which time the horse is likely to have recovered. However, in certain situations a specific diagnosis is beneficial (e.g. in the face of an epidemic, or when a large population of horses is at risk, or if an exotic viral infection is suspected). A variety of laboratory tests for the accurate diagnosis of viral infections is available, and it is recommended that the clinician discusses the requirements for sample collection and submission with an appropriate laboratory beforehand.

The three common methods of diagnosis are as follows.

Serology

A variety of serological tests is used to demonstrate serum antibodies. In most cases, the antibody titres present during the acute stage of the disease need to be compared with those in the convalescent stage 10–14 days later. A fourfold or greater increase in titre is generally considered significant.

Virus isolation

Nasopharyngeal swabs and tracheal aspirates can be used to isolate viruses. Samples need to be taken during the acute phase of disease and it is essential that they are placed immediately into a suitable virus transport medium.

Detection of viral antigens

Viral antigens may be detected in blood, secretions and tissues by a number of techniques which may provide a rapid diagnosis.

Treatment of viral infections

Specific antiviral treatment is rarely used for respiratory viral infections, and prevention through vaccination and management are the main methods of control. Symptomatic therapy is important to prevent long-term sequelae and consideration should be given to the following:

(1)   Rest, to permit the rapid healing of damaged airways. Damage to the mucociliary escalator of the airways can take approximately a month to repair. If the horse is not rested during this period, there is a high probability that airborne dust, microbes and other toxic materials will be retained within the tract, increasing the risk of development of allergy, infections, etc.
(2)   Provision of a clean dust-free environment, to reduce the incidence of post viral bronchopneumonia and COPD (see Chapter 8).
(3)   Antibiotic therapy, if secondary bacterial infection is severe.
(4)   Non-steroidal anti-inflammatory drugs such as phenylbutazone, which may be helpful in horses with high fever or depression.
(5)   Bronchodilators such as clenbuterol (Ventipulmin, Boehringer Ingelheim) and mucolytics such as dembrexine hydrochloride (Sputolosin, Boehringer Ingelheim), which are reported to be beneficial in some cases.

(6)   Immune-stimulating drugs, which are reported to be helpful in viral infections (at present, however, there are no licensed products available in the UK).

STRANGLES

Strangles – infection with *Streptococcus equi* – is highly contagious among susceptible horses. Transmission is either direct (horse-to-horse contact or aerosol) or indirect by way of contaminated buckets, feed, stables, personnel, etc. A carrier state may also arise, which can spread the infection. The initial clinical signs of typical strangles include fever (up to 40 °C/104 °F), depression, anorexia, submandibular lymph node enlargement, slight cough, and a serous nasal discharge which later becomes purulent (Fig. 9.4). The lymph nodes continue to enlarge over the next 7–10 days, and the horse may stand with its head and neck extended because of pain. Usually one or all of the submandibular and retropharyngeal nodes are affected. Dyspnoea and dysphagia may be observed. The abscessed submandibular lymph nodes usually rupture through the skin, and this is followed in most cases by rapid healing and recovery (Fig. 9.5). Potential complications include necrotic pneumonia, metastasis of *S. equi* to other lymph nodes ("bastard strangles"), guttural pouch empyema and purpura haemorrhagica. Diagnosis is usually based on the clinical signs. It can be confirmed by isolation

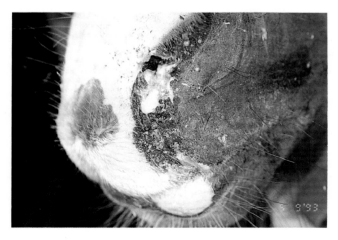

Fig. 9.4 Purulent nasal discharge typical of *S. equi* infection (strangles).

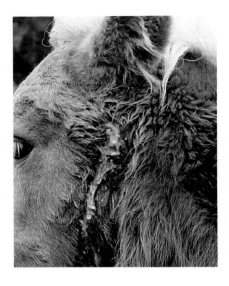

Fig. 9.5 Rupture of abscessed lymph nodes in strangles most commonly occurs in the submandibular area, but can also occur in the parotid region and sometimes elsewhere on the body.

of *S. equi* from an abscess; the organism may be isolated from a nasal swab, although it may be swamped by secondary bacterial invaders such as *Streptococcus zooepidemicus*.

An atypical or catarrhal form of strangles is seen in older horses or in association with a non-encapsulated strain of *S. equi*, and appears to have become commoner in recent years. Atypical strangles is milder, with signs of cough, mild pyrexia, slight nasal discharge and usually only a slight enlargement of the lymph nodes which seldom form abscesses. This form of the disease can be difficult to distinguish clinically from EHV infection in some horses.

Treatment in horses with lymph node abscesses is aimed at enhancing the maturation and drainage of the abscesses. Infected horses should be isolated, and the abscesses lanced if they fail to rupture spontaneously. It is believed that antibiotic therapy administered prior to abscess drainage may simply prolong the course of the disease. Additional therapy that may be indicated in some cases includes feeding by nasogastric tube, tracheostomy and intravenous fluid therapy. Prolonged and aggressive treatment with penicillin is required for horses with bastard strangles. Horses with purpura haemorrhagica require treatment with penicillin and corticosteroids.

Horses exposed to *S. equi* or in the early stage of infection (i.e. within 24 hours of the onset of pyrexia) may be treated with penicillin to prevent the progression of the disease. However, such treatment is likely to prevent the development of protective immunity.

BACTERIAL LOWER RESPIRATORY TRACT INFECTION

Infection of the lower respiratory tract by bacteria, in the absence of a primary viral infection, is a common cause of respiratory disease in young thoroughbred racehorses. In particular, infections with *Streptococcus zooepidemicus*, *S. pneumoniae*, *Pasteurella* spp. and *Mycoplasma* spp. are associated with inflammation of the lower airways. The clinical features of these infections vary from subclinical disease or exercise intolerance in the absence of other clinical signs, to a mild clinical disease characterized by coughing, pyrexia, nasal discharge and enlargement of the submandibular lymph nodes. Tracheal and bronchial exudate is observed endoscopically, and the diagnosis is confirmed by cytological and bacteriological examination of tracheal aspirates or bronchoalveolar lavage samples. Treatment consists of rest, antibiotics and mucolytics, as necessary.

CHOKE, DYSPHAGIA

Any cause of dysphagia can result in the sudden onset of coughing as a result of aspiration of food and saliva into the larynx and trachea. The commonest cause of dysphagia is oesophageal food impaction (choke). Characteristic clinical signs include frequent, unsuccessful attempts to swallow, coughing, ptyalism and nasal return of feed and saliva (Fig. 9.6).

ACUTE AIRWAY OBSTRUCTION

Allergic lower airway diseases – COPD and SPAOPD – are well recognized as causes of chronic coughing (see Chapter 8), but sudden acute onset coughing can also occur, especially in horses exposed to a sudden change in environmental allergens. Typically, acute airway obstruction is seen in horses with a history of COPD that develop respiratory distress within hours of being stabled. A change of diet (especially hay) or bedding, or concur-

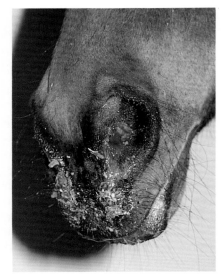

Fig. 9.6 Nasal return of food or saliva is a sign of choke.

rent infection by a virus, may also precipitate an acute attack. Sometimes the disease is seen in horses at grass, in which case exposure to pollens is assumed to be the trigger.

The clinical signs include paroxysmal coughing, dyspnoea and tachypnoea. Auscultation of the lungs usually reveals widespread crackling and wheezing adventitious sounds; crackling sounds are often audible to the naked ear at the nostrils. The horse should be removed from the offending environment to reduce exposure to aeroallergens. Bronchodilator therapy such as clenbuterol (Ventipulmin) is helpful. Corticosteroids such as dexamethasone (10–20 mg) are also useful. In severe cases, rapid bronchodilation may be achieved by using atropine (at 0.015 mg/kg), but its potential side-effects include tachycardia and ileus.

ACUTE PHARYNGITIS AND LARYNGITIS

Inflammation of the pharynx and larynx can arise from a number of causes, the most common being viral infections. Chronic hyperplasia of pharyngeal lymphoid tissue is frequently observed endoscopically in young horses (especially those less than 5 years old), and probably represents a response to novel bacterial and viral infections; this reaction is usually asymptomatic (Fig. 9.7). However, a severe phargyngeal reaction can cause clinical disease. Acute pharyngeal and laryngeal inflammation may also arise secondary to trauma (e.g. from stomach tubing or ingested foreign bodies). On occasion, these reactions may result in clinical signs of coughing, ptyalism, pharyngeal swelling, pain and dysphagia. Treatment is symptomatic.

LUNGWORM

Lungworm infection is discussed in Chapter 8.

EXERCISE-INDUCED PULMONARY HAEMORRHAGE

Exercise-induced pulmonary haemorrhage (EIPH) may occasionally cause coughing after exercise, although it is more commonly associated with poor performance, "gurgling", excessive swallowing and epistaxis. Most racehorses affected by EIPH show no overt clinical signs. The aetiopathogenesis of EIPH is uncertain, although the site of haemorrhage is usually the dorsocaudal lung tips. Diagnosis may be achieved by endoscopic examination of the trachea and bronchi after galloping exercise, or by radiography of the dorsocaudal lung fields.

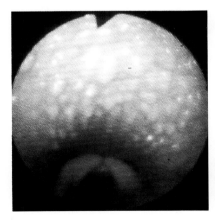

Fig. 9.7 Endoscopic appearance of pharyngeal lymphoid hyperplasia. This hyperplastic lymphoid tissue is commonly observed as a normal finding in young adult horses, and is not usually associated with overt clinical disease.

PLEUROPNEUMONIA, PNEUMONIA, LUNG ABSCESS

Severe bacterial infections of the lung and pleural cavity are uncommon in adult horses in the UK. However, they may be encountered following aspiration of food and saliva (e.g. as a consequence of choke) or in horses stressed by long-distance travel. The onset of disease is often sudden, and is characterized by a variety of signs including fever, tachypnoea and dyspnoea, nasal discharge (Fig. 9.8), cough, pyrexia, thoracic pain and sternal oedema. The infection frequently becomes chronic (see Chapter 8).

Rhodococcus equi is a cause of suppurative bronchopneumonia and lung abscesses in foals, especially those aged 2–6 months. In the UK, the prevalence of *R. equi* pneumonia is low, but the organism can become endemic on certain farms. Dusty environments and dry weather conditions increase the prevalence of the disease. Two clinical forms are recognized. The subacute form is characterized by miliary pyogranulomatous pneumonia, producing clinical signs of severe dyspnoea and tachypnoea, fever and depression; affected foals frequently die within a few days. The chronic form is characterized by less severe respiratory distress, fever and ill-thrift; coughing and nasal discharge are variable features. The diagnosis is based on the clinical features, isolation of *R. equi* from a transtracheal aspirate, and chest radiography. Chest radiographs show a prominent alveolar

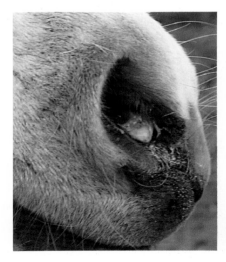

Fig. 9.8 Thick, purulent nasal discharge associated with pneumonia and lung abscesses in a pony. The discharge may be blood-tinged and malodorous.

pattern with regional consolidation; nodular opacities indicative of abscesses are commonly present, and some cases have a pleural effusion.

Treatment involves combined therapy with erythromycin (25 mg/kg orally three times daily) and rifampicin (5 mg/kg orally twice daily). Erythromycin alone may be effective if economics do not justify or permit the use of both drugs. Treatment should be continued for 4–12 weeks until the chest radiology and plasma fibrinogen levels are normal. The prognosis is fair, with approximately 80% of horses recovering after appropriate treatment. The prognosis for future athletic soundness is good.

INHALED FOREIGN BODIES

Foreign bodies may lodge in the nose, pharynx or tracheobronchial tree. Lower airway foreign bodies are usually brambles (Fig. 9.9). The clinical signs include paroxysmal coughing and malodorous breath. Diagnosis is achieved by endoscopy. Removal of the foreign body may require general anaesthesia and tracheotomy.

TRACHEAL COLLAPSE OR CONSTRICTION

Tracheal collapse is occasionally encountered in aged ponies presenting with coughing and adventitious noise. Constriction

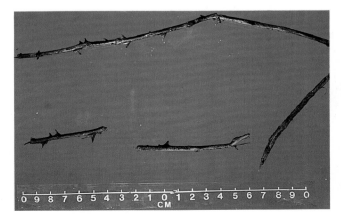

Fig. 9.9 Tracheobronchial foreign body (bramble) removed by snaring via a tracheotomy.

of the tracheal lumen may arise from trauma or may be caused by a congenital defect of the tracheal cartilage rings (Fig. 9.10). The onset of clinical signs is often sudden, even if the lesion is long-standing. Diagnosis is achieved by endoscopy.

RUPTURE OF MITRAL CHORDAE TENDINEAE

Rupture of the mitral chordae tendineae is the most likely cardiac cause of acute onset coughing. The signs include acute respiratory distress and coughing, due to pulmonary oedema, with a widely radiating systolic murmur of mitral regurgitation. Bacterial endocarditis may also present with coughing, usually in conjunction with other signs of disseminated sepsis such as pyrexia, septic arthritis, haematuria and pyuria.

PULMONARY OEDEMA

Pulmonary oedema (Fig. 9.11) is rarely encountered in adult horses, but may arise as a life-threatening complication of other conditions, such as smoke inhalation, acute renal failure, overhydration, septicaemia and anaphylaxis. The clinical signs include dyspnoea (rapid shallow respirations), coughing, fluid discharge from the nose (which may be blood-tinged or frothy), distress, cyanosis, collapse and death. Treatment is aimed at correcting the underlying cause, in addition to the administration of diuretics.

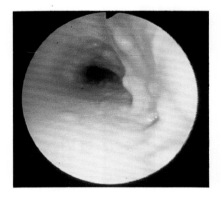

Fig. 9.10 Tracheal cartilage deformity resulting in luminal constriction, as seen endoscopically. The clinical signs, including cough and adventitious noise, may have a sudden onset.

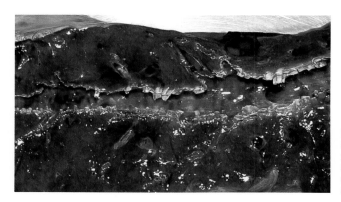

Fig. 9.11 Post-mortem appearance of pulmonary oedema secondary to septicaemia in an adult horse.

FURTHER READING

Beech, J. (1991) *Equine Respiratory Disorders*. Lea & Febiger, Philadelphia.

Churnside, E. D. (1993) Equine viral arteritis – a free market threat. *Equine Veterinary Education* **5**, 137–139.

Robertson, J. T. & Reed, S. M. (1991) Respiratory disease: medicine and surgery. *Veterinary Clinics of North America (Equine Practice)* **7** (1).

Traub-Dargatz, J. L. (1993) Update on infectious diseases. *Veterinary Clinics of North America (Equine Practice)* **9** (2).

CHAPTER 10

Management of Oesophageal Obstruction (Choke)

MARK HILLYER

Oesophageal disorders (Table 10.1) are relatively uncommon in the horse in comparison with other domesticated species. However, because of their dramatic and acute presentation, they often cause the owner considerable concern and anxiety. This chapter outlines the aetiology, diagnosis and treatment of oesophageal obstructions in horses.

CAUSES OF OESOPHAGEAL OBSTRUCTION

The commonest equine oesophageal condition is simple obstruction (choke). Usually this is a primary problem caused

Table 10.1 Potential oesophageal disorders in the horse.

Oesophageal obstruction – "choke"
Oesophageal ulceration
Oesophageal stricture
Oesophageal neoplasia
Oesophageal perforation/rupture
Oesophageal compression by external tissues
Megaoesophagus
Oesophageal diverticulum
Congenital/developmental oesophageal abnormalities

Table 10.2 Potential causes of primary oesophageal obstruction in the horse.

Improperly soaked sugarbeet

Hay, bedding

Grass cubes, commercial cubes

Corn cobs

Specific foreign body:
  twig(s)
  bramble(s)
  wood, wood chips, bark
  fragment(s) of nasogastric tubing
  wire/metallic body
  medication bolus

---

by the attempted ingestion of inappropriate material (Table 10.2). The feeding of inadequately soaked sugarbeet pulp or inadvertent access to dry sugarbeet pulp are the most common causes. Other causes include too rapid ingestion of dry fibrous material (e.g. hay), inadequate mastication of feed due to poor dentition, or the swallowing of a foreign body; these are, however, less common as horses are usually slow and discriminate feeders.

Oesophageal obstruction may also be seen as a secondary feature of other oesophageal conditions (Table 10.3). In these cases, the absence of a history of ingestion of an unsuitable material, a poor response to treatment or the occurrence of repeated

Table 10.3 Conditions that may lead to the development of a secondary oesophageal obstruction.

Oesophageal ulceration/oesophagitis

Oesophageal stricture

Megaoesophagus

Oesophageal neoplasia

Space-occupying masses causing oesophageal compression

Oesophageal diverticulum

Oesophageal cysts/other congenital anomalies

Table 10.4 Clinical signs that may be associated with oesophageal obstruction.

Dysphagia

Drooling of saliva

Nasal return of saliva or food (immediate or delayed)

Visible or palpable mass on left lateroventral aspect of neck

Repeated attempts at swallowing

Repeated arching or spasm of neck muscles

Marked anxiety or distress

Coughing

Pyrexia

Halitosis

---

episodes of choke should alert the attending clinician to the possibility of a separate underlying primary oesophageal lesion.

CLINICAL SIGNS

The clinical signs shown will vary from case to case depending on the nature, site and extent of the oesophageal obstruction and its duration (Table 10.4). Typically, the major sign is dysphagia with nasal return of food and saliva (Fig. 10.1). It may

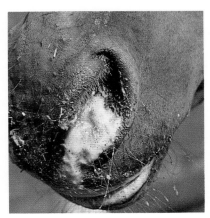

Fig. 10.1 Nasal return of food and saliva in a horse with an oesophageal obstruction.

M. H. Hillyer

occur during attempted swallowing, immediately after feeding or several hours later, and this variation may be indicative of the site of the obstruction along the length of the oesophagus. If the site of the obstruction leads to accumulation of material in the cervical oesophagus then a visible or palpable mass may be apparent on the left ventrolateral aspect of the neck (Fig. 10.2). Unlike cases of secondary oesophageal obstruction, which may have an insidious onset, most cases of primary choke are acute in nature with a sudden onset of signs related to the complete obstruction of the oesophagus. The presence of pyrexia and halitosis are usually indicative of the development of a secondary aspiration pneumonia.

In long-standing cases of choke, further signs may develop related to the persistent loss of saliva and failure of water and nutrient intake. These include dehydration, electrolyte and acid–base disturbances and weight loss.

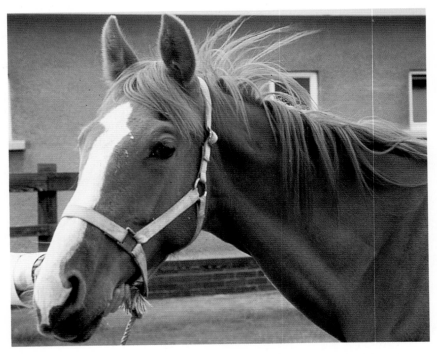

Fig. 10.2 Oesophageal obstruction in a horse with a visible mass on the left ventrolateral aspect of the neck.

DIAGNOSIS

A diagnosis of oesophageal obstruction may be suspected from the presence of typical clinical signs (Table 10.4) and an appropriate history of access to an unsuitable feed. Some other potential causes of dysphagia in the horse are listed in Table 10.5 and these should be considered in cases of dysphagia where an initial suspicion of an oesophageal obstruction is not confirmed.

The diagnosis may be confirmed by the presence of an obstruction to the passage of a nasogastric tube. Care must be taken not to exert excessive force with the nasogastric tube – forced pulsion of the impaction is rarely successful and carries a considerable risk of causing further damage to the oesophagus itself. The level of the rostral end of the obstruction may also be determined from the length of tube which can be passed, although the position of the distal limit will not be ascertained. Further confirmatory procedures include endoscopic and radiographic examination of the oesophagus (Figs 10.3–5). Oesophagoscopy may be performed with a 1.2 m gastroscope, but for visualization of the entire oesophagus a longer endoscope (up to 2.5 m) is required. Oesophagoscopy will usually determine the rostral limit of the obstruction and may give some information as to its nature. However, the presence of secondarily impacted food material and saliva may prevent visualization of a foreign body or primary oesophageal lesion. In these

Table 10.5 Common causes of dysphagia in the horse.

Oesophageal obstruction

Dental abnormalities

Guttural pouch disease

Oral/pharyngeal foreign body

Grass sickness

Palatal defects

Botulism

Lead poisoning

Tetanus

(A)

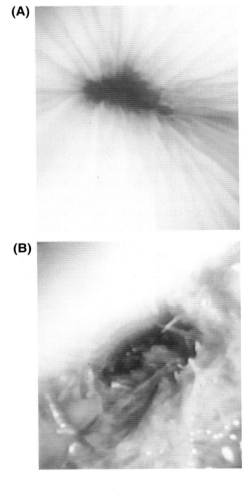

(B)

Fig. 10.3 Endoscopic view of a normal equine oesophagus (A) and the oesophagus of a horse with a feed impaction (B).

cases, radiography, prior to attempted treatment of the impaction, may be more rewarding. Standing lateral views of the cervical and thoracic oesophagus are the most useful. These may be enhanced by the use of positive or negative contrast agents to delineate further the oesophagus. In cases where endoscopy reveals a specific foreign body as the cause of the obstruction, endoscopic removal under direct visualization may be attempted.

The use of endoscopy also allows inspection of the trachea for evidence of aspiration of food material or saliva into the

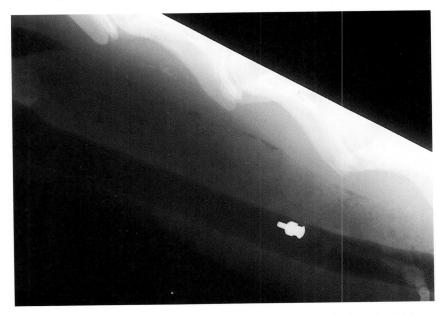

Fig. 10.4 Radiograph of the cervical oesophagus of a pony with a primary oesophageal feed impaction. A delivery apparatus for the administration of intravenous fluids is also visible.

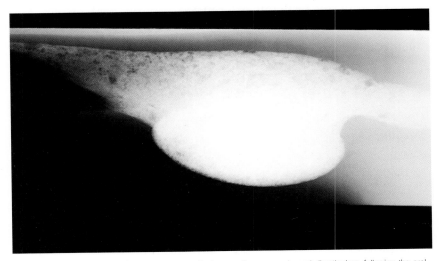

Fig. 10.5 Radiograph of the cervical oesophagus of a horse with an oesophageal diverticulum, following the oral administration of a barium suspension.

airway. The presence of foreign materials in the trachea is a common and potentially serious complication of oesophageal choke and can lead to the development of a secondary inhalation pneumonia. This can be monitored by careful thoracic auscultation and at least daily monitoring of the rectal temperature, combined with cytology and culture of any airway discharge, haematology, thoracic radiography or thoracic ultrasonography, as deemed appropriate.

TREATMENT

The initial treatment of oesophageal choke is conservative, as many obstructions will resolve spontaneously or with medical management. However, in all cases of suspected oesophageal choke, including those in which apparent spontaneous resolution has occurred, the possibility of inhalation pneumonia should be assessed and appropriate antimicrobial therapy instituted where necessary. This would usually entail the administration of a broad-spectrum, bactericidal antimicrobial agent or a suitable combination of agents (Table 10.6).

The medical treatment of oesophageal choke usually comprises the use of sedatives to reduce the anxiety of the horse, smooth muscle relaxants to reduce oesophageal spasm and

Table 10.6 Antimicrobial agents which may be used in cases of oesophageal choke with suspected aspiration of foreign material into the lower airway.

Drug	Dose	Route and frequency
Crystalline penicillin	10 000–50 000 iu/kg	IV, four times daily
Procaine penicillin	20 000–50 000 iu/kg	IM, twice daily
Gentamicin	2–4 mg/kg	IV, twice daily
Streptomycin	11 mg/kg	IM, once daily
Potentiated sulphonamides	30 mg/kg	IV, once daily
Metronidazole	15 mg/kg	PO, three times daily
Ceftiofur	2 mg/kg	IM, once daily

NB – These drugs are not necessarily licensed for this use in the horse.
IV, intravenously; IM, intramuscularly; PO, by mouth.

allow passage of the impacted material, analgesics to reduce oesophageal pain and anti-inflammatory agents to control the oesophageal inflammation. These goals can be achieved by the use of one or a combination of several therapeutic agents, and examples are listed in Table 10.7. If the use of these agents is not successful in allowing the obstruction to clear then they may be repeated or alternative agents tried once the effects of the initial treatment have worn off. In practice, this usually involves repeating the medical treatment at intervals of 8–12 hours. During this time the horse should be denied access to food or water to reduce the risk of aspiration of foreign material into the trachea. Care, however, should be taken with the concurrent intravenous use of potentiated sulphonamides and detomidine.

More aggressive treatment for choke involves oesophageal lavage (see below) in an attempt to soften and break down the impaction. This technique carries a small but increased risk of inadvertent aspiration of foreign material into the lower airways and hence would usually be reserved for cases in which initial medical management was not successful. In such cases, it is likely to be used 24–48 hours after the onset of the impaction.

Table 10.7 Drugs which may be used in the medical management of oesophageal choke.

Drug	Intravenous dose (mg/kg)
For sedation/oesophageal relaxation	
Acepromazine	0.05
Xylazine	0.5–1
Detomidine	0.01–0.02
Romifidine	0.04–0.12
For oesophageal muscle relaxation/analgesia/ anti-inflammatory effect	
Hyoscine:dipyrone	0.5:22
For analgesia/anti-inflammatory effect	
Flunixin	1.1
Phenylbutazone	2.4
For analgesia	
Butorphanol	0.5–2

NB – These drugs are not necessarily licensed for this use in the horse.

Where a specific foreign body is suspected to be present from the history or clinical, endoscopic or radiographic examination, removal via an endoscope may be possible. This technique requires the foreign body to be visible endoscopically and also amenable to grasping by suitable forceps or snare. This may not be possible until the surrounding feed impaction has been removed by prior oesophageal lavage.

In a few cases, conservative management is unsuccessful, necessitating surgical removal. There are several reports of surgical techniques for oesophagotomy in the horse, but as these would usually be performed at a specialist referral centre they are not discussed further here. Oesophageal surgery is not without its complications (e.g. wound dehiscence, cellulitis and oesophageal stricture formation) and these would need to be considered prior to surgery.

OTHER CONSIDERATIONS

The presence of an oesophageal obstruction will invariably be associated with a failure of water intake. In addition, the inability to swallow saliva will lead to further losses of fluid and electrolytes. In acute cases (up to 24 hours' duration), this does not normally represent a clinical problem and, following resolution of the impaction, oral fluid intake will rapidly allow correction of any deficits. In chronic cases (over 48 hours' duration), any degree of dehydration or electrolyte/acid–base imbalance needs to be determined and treated accordingly. Equine saliva contains high concentrations of sodium and chloride and hence most cases of choke provoke hyponatraemia and hypochloraemia. The acid–base status can, however, be extremely variable and specific treatment is not usually justified without access to blood gas analysis equipment. For most cases where the duration of the impaction has led to dehydration and electrolyte imbalances, treatment with intravenous polyionic fluids is sufficient.

OESOPHAGEAL LAVAGE TECHNIQUE

Oesophageal lavage may be performed in the standing animal or with the horse in lateral recumbency under general anaesthesia.

In the standing horse

In the standing horse the risk of aspiration of foreign material is greater. This risk may be minimized by the use of profound sedation to maintain the horse's head and neck in a lowered position (Fig. 10.6) and, if necessary, the use of a cuffed nasotracheal tube. Lavage is performed through a nasogastric tube inserted to the rostral limit of the impaction. Warm water is then flushed through the tube with the use of a stomach pump. At the same time the tube may be gently manipulated against the impaction.

The returning water and impacted material will emerge out of the mouth and external nares. This effluent should be inspected to try to identify the cause of the impaction. Intermittent, manual external occlusion of the oesophagus rostral to the impaction may be useful to distend the oesophageal wall away from the impaction. If possible, the use of a nasogastric tube with an 'end only' opening is preferable to one with side and end openings so that the majority of the water flow is directed at the impaction. Once the impaction clears, the remaining material is usually flushed into the stomach and the nasogastric tube can then be easily passed to the stomach.

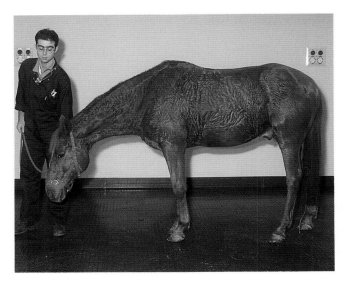

Fig. 10.6 Horse suitably sedated prior to standing oesophageal lavage, with the head and neck lowered to minimize the risk of aspiration.

In the recumbent horse

The technique of oesophageal lavage is similar in the recumbent horse. Once general anaesthesia has been induced, a cuffed endotracheal tube is essential to maintain an airway and prevent aspiration of foreign material. The horse should be positioned in right lateral recumbency with the head and neck lower than the thoracic inlet. The stomach tube may be inserted via the nose or mouth. The latter has the advantage of allowing a wider bore tube to be used and eliminates the possibility of haemorrhage from the nasal passages. However, care is necessary to ensure that this tube passes down the oesophagus and not down the trachea alongside the endotracheal tube. Flushing proceeds in a similar manner to that in the standing horse. Once the impaction has been dispersed, recovery from anaesthesia is routine. However, it is usual to take out the endotracheal tube before the cuff is completely deflated so that any foreign material in the upper trachea is also removed.

Lavage under general anaesthesia will usually produce better oesophageal relaxation than in the standing animal and will allow a larger volume of water to be used safely. General anaesthesia may also allow manual removal of a rostral oesophageal impaction or foreign body via the oropharynx.

SUBSEQUENT MANAGEMENT

Following the clearance of an oesophageal impaction, careful dietary management is essential. Even after short-term, self-resolving chokes, a gradual return to a normal diet is sensible. Initially, this will usually involve access to oral fluids only, followed by the reintroduction of wet, soft feeds (e.g. wet bran mash and gruel). These can be made progressively firmer and drier and then long-fibre forage (e.g. hay or horsehage) may also be included. This progression from oral fluids to a normal diet may take 2–3 days in straightforward cases or as long as 4–6 weeks in chronically obstructed cases with extensive oesophageal damage.

Endoscopy is particularly useful after the impaction has cleared, at which stage a thorough examination of the oesophagus can be performed. Careful observation as the endoscope is passed along the oesophagus will usually allow the site of the previous impaction to be identified. In acute mild cases this may be seen as a localized area of inflammation, but in more severe cases mucosal ulceration may be apparent. In cases where a primary underlying oesophageal lesion is suspected, post-treatment oesophagoscopy is essential for its identification. Once the endoscope has been passed to the stomach, or as far as its length will allow, it should be withdrawn slowly. Further observation at this time, with accompanying inflation of the oesophagus, usually gives the best visualization of the oeso-phageal wall. Recordings of any lesions seen, particularly areas of ulceration, can be useful for comparing with subsequent images in order to assess the healing process and the possible development of an oesophageal stricture.

COMPLICATIONS FOLLOWING OESOPHAGEAL OBSTRUCTION

OESOPHAGEAL INFLAMMATION

Following an oesophageal obstruction, there is inevitably an inflammatory response at the site of the impaction. The extent of the inflammation is normally directly related to the duration of the obstruction. In mild cases this will usually present as a focal area of oesophagitis which is rapidly self-resolving. More severe cases may benefit from the use of non-steroidal anti-inflammatory agents.

OESOPHAGEAL ULCERATION OR STRICTURE FORMATION

Mucosal ulceration is often seen as a sequel to more long-stand-ing cases of oesophageal impaction. Small focal or longitudinal areas of ulceration will usually heal without complications once the original impaction has been cleared (Fig. 10.7). However, the presence of an area of circumferential full-thickness mucosal ulceration is of more concern owing to the association of stric-ture development with the healing of these lesions (Fig. 10.8). In these cases, a slow return to a normal diet is essential to prevent recurrent impactions. Significant stricture formation, and subsequent narrowing of the oesophageal lumen, usually

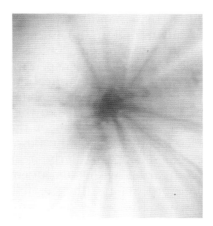

Fig. 10.7 Endoscopic view of the oesophagus of a horse after clearance of a primary feed impaction, showing focal areas of mucosal ulceration.

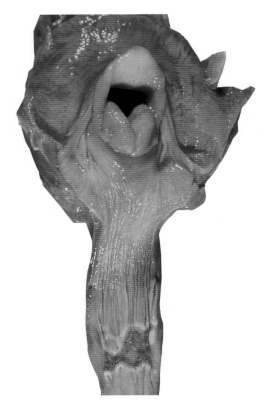

Fig. 10.8 Post-mortem specimen from a foal with an oesophageal obstruction, showing an area of circumferential mucosal ulceration.

develops within 2 weeks and reaches a maximum by 5 weeks after the original impaction. Thereafter, there is usually a period of improvement, with an increase in the oesophageal lumen, for a further 4–5 weeks. During this time the feeding of increasingly bulky food may help to produce a bougienage effect and encourage stretching of the stricture. Subsequently (9–10 weeks after the original impaction), there is usually no further improvement in the extent of the stricture. At this point, careful dietary management is sufficient in most cases to prevent recurrent choke episodes. However, in severe cases surgical intervention may be attempted using a modified oesophagomyotomy or resection of the stricture.

The use of pharmacological agents, such as corticosteroids and colchicine, to prevent stricture formation has been advocated in cases of circumferential ulceration but there is little evidence as to their efficacy.

OESOPHAGEAL PERFORATION

Oesophageal perforation may occur as a result of external trauma to the neck, internal trauma from a foreign body or excessive manipulations with a stomach tube, or ischaemic damage to the oesophageal wall following a chronic impaction. The clinical signs are variable but usually relate to a cellulitis of the perioesophageal tissues, often with associated subcutaneous emphysema; occasionally a cutaneous fistula may develop. Primary surgical repair may be attempted, but in most cases healing by secondary intention is sufficient. Supportive treatments may include feeding via a nasogastric or oesophagotomy tube, antimicrobial therapy and local drainage of the affected tissues. Mediastinitis or pleuritis are potential complications and carry a very poor prognosis.

ASPIRATION PNEUMONIA AND PLEUROPNEUMONIA

The development of a secondary pneumonia or pleuropneumonia is a potential complication of any oesophageal obstruction which causes aspiration of foreign material into the lower airways. Fortunately, only a mild, subclinical pneumonia develops in most cases and this rapidly resolves once the obstruction is cleared and the aspiration stops. However, in some cases with prolonged aspiration, or aspiration of excessive amounts of foreign material, a severe pneumonia or pleuro-pneumonia may develop. The diagnosis of this complication is based on the clinical signs, clinicopathological data and thoracic radiography and ultrasonography. Once the primary choke is resolved, treatment is based on antimicrobial therapy, directed by the results of culture and sensitivity of a sample obtained by airway aspiration or thoracocentesis. Despite this and other supportive treatment, the prognosis for cases that develop secondary pneumonia or pleuropneumonia is guarded.

Acknowledgements

The author would like to thank Dr F. J. Barr, Dr C. Gibbs and Mr J. G. Lane for providing some of the illustrations.

FURTHER READING

Craig, D. R., Shivy, D. R., Pankowski, R. L. & Erb, H. N. (1989) Esophageal disorders in 61 horses: results of nonsurgical and surgical management. *Veterinary Surgery* **18**, 432–438.
Green, E. M. (1992) Esophageal obstruction. In *Current Therapy in Equine Medicine*, vol 3 (ed. N. E. Robinson) pp. 175–184. W. B. Saunders, Philadelphia.
Todhunter, R. J., Stick, J. A., Trotter, G. W. & Boles, C. (1984) Medical management of esophageal stricture in seven horses. *Journal of the American Veterinary Medical Association* **185**, 784–787.

CHAPTER 11

Differential Diagnosis of Gastric Dilatation

BARRIE EDWARDS

The stomach of an adult horse can accommodate as much as 30 litres of fluid, but the dangers of such distension, if prolonged, are rupture or neuromuscular damage to the stomach wall causing atony. The peculiar anatomy of the cardiac region, with its powerful lower oesophageal sphincter which does not yield to increasing intragastric pressure, precludes regurgitation or vomition and often leads to gastric rupture. Most of the reflexes controlling gastric emptying are inhibitory except for distension which stimulates gastric mechanoreceptors. The primary inhibitory control of gastric emptying is the enterogastric reflex initiated by receptors in the duodenum.

Gastric reflux is a not uncommon clinical finding in horses with colic, and differentiation between the various conditions in which it may be a feature is not always straightforward. The accumulation of large volumes of fluid in the stomach may be due to primary gastric dilatation; gastric dilatation secondary to intestinal obstruction; or a functional disturbance due to ileus from a variety of causes (Table 11.1).

PRIMARY GASTRIC DILATATION

Primary gastric dilatation may result from overeating of readily fermentable foodstuffs such as fresh grass or, particularly, grain.

Table 11.1 Causes of gastric dilatation.

Primary gastric dilatation	e.g. grain overload
Small intestinal obstruction	Simple obstruction, e.g. ileal impaction Strangulating obstruction, e.g. epiploic foramen incarceration
Large intestinal obstruction	e.g. left dorsal displacement of the large colon
Ileus	Anterior enteritis Grass sickness Peritonitis Postoperative ileus

Large amounts of starch are not natural in the diet of horses and the considerable amounts of volatile fatty acids produced by the action of the gastric flora on grain inhibits gastric emptying, thereby promoting further fermentation. In addition, there is an associated influx of fluid into the stomach. Shock and metabolic acidosis develop rapidly.

The consumption of large quantities of cold water by a horse soon after exertion may result in pyloric spasm and accompanying gastric dilatation, but this is often transient.

INTESTINAL OBSTRUCTION

Intestinal obstruction causes small intestinal contents to reflux into the stomach where they accumulate and produce distension. The small intestine obstruction may be simple, as in ileal impaction, or strangulating, due to one of a wide variety of causes. Although the obstruction may be located anywhere along the length of the small intestine, obstructions most frequently involve the more distal gut, particularly the ileum. However, proximal obstructions do occur; caused, for example, by stricture secondary to chronic pyloroduodenal ulceration in young thoroughbreds and associated with acute pancreatitis (Fig. 11.1). Gastric reflux may also accompany large colon obstructions, particularly left dorsal displacement (nephrosplenic entrapment) in which secondary impaction in the ventral colon rostral to the nephrosplenic ligament com-

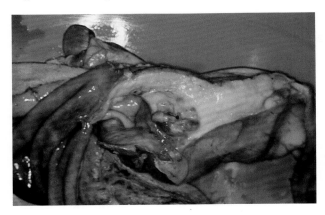

Fig. 11.1 Gross fibrosis of the pylorus and proximal duodenum in a yearling thoroughbred secondary to gastroduodenal ulceration.

presses the duodenum (Fig. 11.2). Consequently, in these cases, decompression of the stomach by nasogastric intubation should always be carried out before inducing general anaesthesia.

More rarely, non-strangulating infarction of the small intestine can be the cause of gastric dilatation.

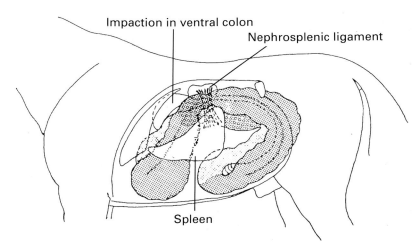

Impaction in ventral colon

Nephrosplenic ligament

Spleen

Fig. 11.2 Left dorsal displacement of the large colon. The secondary impaction in the ventral colon cranial to the nephrosplenic ligament often obstructs the small intestine, leading to gastric dilatation.

ILEUS

ANTERIOR (PROXIMAL) ENTERITIS

The term "anterior enteritis" is used to describe an acute clinical syndrome characterized by abdominal pain, ileus, gastric distension and hypovolaemic shock, often complicated by endotoxic shock. This relatively new intestinal disease involving the duodenum and proximal jejunum was first recognized in Georgia, U.S.A., in 1977. It was subsequently seen with increasing frequency throughout the United States and parts of Canada. Huskamp reported the condition in West Germany in 1981 and the author encountered the condition for the first time in the UK in 1984.

The disease can only be diagnosed definitively at surgery or necropsy, but in most cases the signs are said to be specific enough to allow a clinical diagnosis to be made.

Clinical signs

Horses present with moderate to severe colic accompanied frequently by marked sweating. Depression may replace the colic after 12–24 hours although most horses continue to show intermittent pain. Ileus is a consistent physical finding. Gastric distension occurs secondary to the ileus, hypersecretion and decreased absorption of fluid within a few hours of the onset of the condition and, in extreme cases, may result in some stomach contents being expelled via the nose. The volume of gastroenteric fluid obtained on nasogastric intubation varies from 5 litres to 30 litres. The fluid is usually fetid, alkaline and brownish tinged. It frequently contains occult blood.

Many horses have a fever and an accompanying leucocytosis. Varying degrees of dehydration and endotoxic shock are seen. Heart rate (70–100/min) and respiratory rate (30–60/min) are elevated and capillary refill time is extended to 4–6 seconds. Mucous membranes are congested and injected and, in cases presented in severe shock, are cyanotic. Usually there are no intestinal borborygmi evident on abdominal auscultation. Laminitis is a not infrequent complication in horses that survive the initial acute phase of the disease.

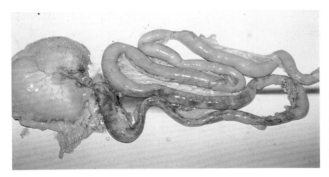

Fig. 11.3 Appearance of proximal small intestine in anterior enteritis; the serosal surface shows patchy yellow and haemorrhagic discoloration.

Findings at laparotomy or necropsy

At laparotomy or necropsy varying lengths of the proximal small intestine are found to be moderately distended, but its diameter is rarely greater than 7 cm and the intraluminal pressure is usually less than 10 cmH$_2$O. The serosal surface of the duodenum and proximal jejunum has streaks of petechial haemorrhage and pale yellow lymphatics; in some cases large areas of ecchymotic haemorrhage are present (Figs 11.3, 11.4). The wall of the affected gut is slightly thickened but is not as oedematous as infarcted or obstructed intestine. In some cases, the lesions may progress to focal necrosis of the intestinal wall. Haemorrhages may also be seen in the mesoduodenum and mesojejunum together with subserosal oedema at the junction

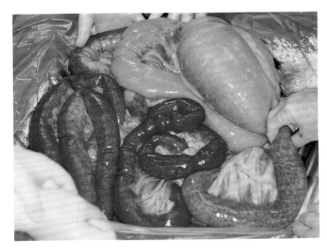

Fig. 11.4 Anterior enteritis; the small intestine shows large areas of ecchymotic haemorrhage.

of the mesentery and intestine. The rest of the small intestine is contracted.

Histology

The histological lesions are confined to the duodenum and proximal jejunum in most cases, but can extend from the stomach to the colon. There is submucosal and mucosal oedema, and hyperaemia with sloughing of the villous epithelium. In severe lesions there is neutrophilic infiltration and degeneration in the submucosa, together with haemorrhages in the muscularis and submucosa. The severity of the lesions varies between cases.

The disease in Germany also has an associated haemorrhagic gastritis which is not commonly encountered in cases seen in the UK and the USA.

Aetiology

The aetiology of anterior enteritis is unknown. *Clostridium* and *Salmonella* species have been suggested as possible causes. The histological lesion is similar to clostridial enteritis in young pigs, but is unlike the recognized clostridial enteritis in the horse which usually produces lesions in the caecum and colon. However, in 14 of 26 horses presented to the author in which gastric or intestinal contents were cultured, *Clostridium perfringens* was isolated (Edwards, 1992).

GRASS SICKNESS

Grass sickness is a non-infectious dysautonomic disease of Equidae of unknown origin which appears to be restricted in occurrence to the UK and other European countries. There is no breed or sex predisposition and any age of horse other than suckling foals may be affected; the condition, however, is seen most frequently in horses between 2 years and 7 years of age. Cases may be seen throughout the year but the highest incidence is in the late spring and early summer. As the name suggests, grass sickness is seen in horses which are at pasture at least part of the time. Mortality rates are very high and only some chronic cases with the least damage to intrinsic intestinal nerve supply can be nursed to recovery.

Grass sickness occurs in peracute, acute, subacute and chronic forms, all of which are generally regarded as representing differing degrees in the manifestation of one pathological condition. Gastric dilatation is usually restricted to the peracute and acute forms where there is virtually complete bowel stasis. The grossly distended stomach may contain in excess of 30 litres of fluid and gastric rupture is not uncommon. Abdominal pain, which can be severe, may be accompanied by patchy sweating and fine muscular tremors. Drooling of saliva is another common feature of the disease. The condition is essentially a neurogenic obstruction affecting different parts of the alimentary tract to varying degrees.

ADYNAMIC ILEUS

Adynamic ileus may be caused by severe peritonitis but is most commonly found in postoperative colic cases. It is characterized by lack of borborygmi and by sequestration of fluid in the intestine and stomach resulting in large volumes of gastric reflux.

CLINICAL SIGNS OF GASTRIC DILATATION

The most consistent clinical sign of gastric dilatation is abdominal pain. The severity of pain and clinical deterioration is proportional to the severity and duration of the dilatation. Primary gastric dilatation usually presents as acute colic. Abdominal distension is not seen because of the position of the stomach within the rib cage, but dyspnoea may be evident due to pressure on the diaphragm. In cases of secondary gastric dilatation the clinical signs are often dependent upon the primary intestinal lesion. In addition to various manifestations of pain, clinical signs include increased heart and respiratory rates, sweating and depression. Abnormal postures such as "dog-sitting" are frequently described but rarely observed.

Although eructation or the presence of small amounts of ingesta at the nostrils may indicate severe gastric distension, its diagnosis in the majority of cases is dependent upon the passage of a nasogastric tube and the subsequent reflux of a significant volume of gastric fluid and gas (Fig. 11.5). This underlines the importance of carrying out the procedure routinely in horses with colic. When the distended stomach is entered gastric fluid usually flows spontaneously. However, the tube may require repositioning to locate pockets of fluid. Aspiration and initiation of a siphon by administering small volumes of water may be necessary to initiate flow. The fluid should be collected in one or more buckets so that a fairly accurate estimation of the total volume can be obtained.

It is important not to abandon attempts to obtain reflux until several minutes have been spent repeatedly repositioning the end of the tube and applying suction.

GASTRIC RUPTURE

If a horse is observed to retch or vomit, it is usually a terminal event associated with gastric rupture. The rupture is generally located on a line parallel with the greater curvature and about 5 cm medial to it (Figs 11.6, 11.7). The ingesta is initially trapped in the omentum but is quickly disseminated throughout the abdomen resulting in a fulminating peritonitis which is rapidly fatal. Characteristically, a horse with gastric rupture is severely depressed and stands immobile because of severe parietal pain (Fig. 11.8). Rigid "boarding" of the abdominal musculature is

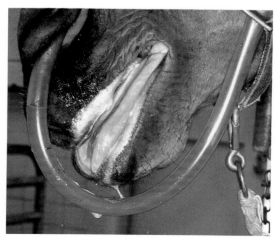

Fig. 11.5 Horse with nasogastric tube in situ. Reflux fluid can be seen in the tube.

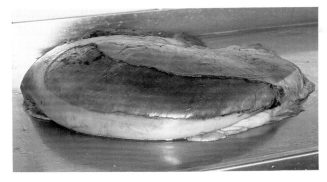

Fig. 11.6 Rupture of the stomach along the greater curvature. In this case there was a long seromuscular tear with only a small hole in the mucosa which had led to a large volume of gastric fluid escaping into the peritoneal cavity.

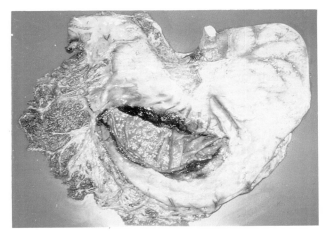

Fig. 11.7 Gastric rupture. Extensive tear through all layers.

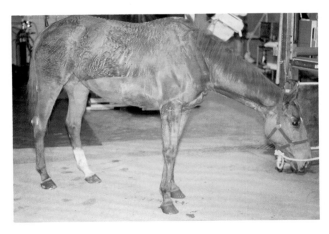

Fig. 11.8 Horse with gastric rupture; it is severely depressed, standing motionless and sweating profusely.

further evidence of the intense parietal peritoneal inflammation. The heart rate is in excess of 100 per minute and the pulse is weak and difficult to palpate. The horse sweats profusely but its extremities are cold. Respirations are rapid and shallow, and the mucous membranes are cyanotic. The horse succumbs rapidly to overwhelming shock.

DIFFERENTIAL DIAGNOSIS OF GASTRIC DILATATION

Aids to the differential diagnosis of gastric dilatation include:

(1)   History.
(2)   Effect of decompression.
(3)   Examination of gastric fluid.
(4)   Rectal examination.
(5)   Examination of peritoneal fluid.
(6)   Laparotomy.

HISTORY

As in all cases of colic, it is essential to determine as accurately as possible the time that has elapsed since the onset of abdominal pain. Without this information it is difficult to evaluate the significance of clinical findings. Whereas reflux of significant volumes of intestinal fluid into the stomach will not occur until many hours after obstruction of the distal small intestine, gross gastric distension may be present within a very few hours of the onset of primary dilatation or anterior enteritis. A history of unlimited access to grain may help to identify primary gastric dilatation. The time of the year, age of the horse and the fact that it is at pasture may point to grass sickness as a likely cause. Additional aids to the diagnosis of grass sickness include:

(1)   Radiography and barium studies of oesophageal dysfunction.
(2)   Measurement of plasma catecholamines.
(3)   Evaluation of gut neuropeptides.
(4)   The definitive diagnosis has been identification of neurological degeneration in the cranial mesenteric or other sympathetic ganglia.

(5) Confirmation is now possible on histological examination of an ileal biopsy.

EFFECT OF DECOMPRESSION

Gastric decompression in primary dilatation should produce a marked improvement and effect a cure if secondary complications such as laminitis and gastric rupture have not occurred. In contrast, if the dilatation is secondary to small intestinal obstruction, decompression of the stomach will only partially and temporarily alleviate the problem.

EXAMINATION OF GASTRIC FLUID

The colour of gastric reflux is variable and not a reliable indication of its underlying cause. Stomach contents are normally green, relatively sweet-smelling and have a pH in the range 3 to 6 (Table 11.2). If reflux has occurred from the small intestine the fluid is yellow/brown, but a subjective impression of biliary reflux on the basis of colour is not a reliable criterion. Red/brown discoloration due to the presence of occult blood is highly suggestive of anterior enteritis but it is not a constant feature and may occasionally be seen in conjunction with duodenal infarction or strangulating obstruction of the proximal jejunum. The reflux in anterior enteritis and in horses with physical obstructions of the small intestine is usually alkaline

Table 11.2 Gastric fluid as a diagnostic aid.

	Colour	Odour	pH
Normal	Green	Relatively sweet	3–6
Small intestinal obstruction	Yellow/brown	Fetid	6–8
Anterior enteritis	May be red/brown owing to occult blood	Fetid	6–8
Grass sickness	Green	Fetid	6–8

(pH 6 to 8) owing to the buffering effects of intestinal fluid. However, a high pH is equally unreliable evidence of intestinal reflux because the pH of gastric fluid can vary widely in the absence of normal stimuli.

RECTAL EXAMINATION

The presence of distended loops of small intestine suggests that gastric dilatation is secondary to intestinal obstruction – physical or functional. Taken in conjunction with the duration of the symptoms the rectal findings (Fig. 11.9) will help to identify the likely site of the obstruction. Multiple distended loops filling the caudal abdomen, together with a large volume of gastric reflux, are consistent with obstruction of the distal small intestine, but such generalized distension is also present in acute grass sickness and idiopathic ileus. The absence of rectal abnormalities with no palpable distension of the small intestine, combined with gastric distension, indicates a high small intestinal or pyloric obstruction, or a gastric problem. Duodenal disease is similar unless the problem is just distal to the duodenum when the moderately distended duodenum can be palpated over the base of the caecum; this, together with one or two loops of distended jejunum, is a common finding in anterior enteritis.

In grass sickness the large colon is contracted down on to firm digesta giving it a corrugated form, rather than the smoothly distended form characteristic of a primary impaction. However, similar contraction of the colon is also seen in horses with

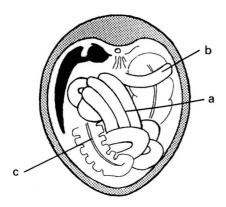

Fig. 11.9 Summary of rectal findings: (a) distended loops of jejunum; (b) distended duodenum; (c) large colon contracted down on dry, impacted contents.

anterior enteritis and ileal impaction resulting from absorption of water to compensate for the loss of fluid sequestered in the stomach and small intestine.

Left dorsal displacement and other colonic problems which occasionally are accompanied by gastric reflux are easily identified.

EXAMINATION OF PERITONEAL FLUID

Peritoneal fluid analysis is not a definitive test for diagnosing the acute abdomen but it is a sensitive indicator of bowel injury (Table 11.3). Peritoneal fluid may be evaluated by gross visual examination, total protein determination and microscopic evaluation. Normal peritoneal fluid is yellow and clear, with no red blood cells and less than 5000 white blood cells per ml. It changes with specific disease, becoming more turbid as a result of increases in protein, red blood cells and leucocytes.

Serosanguineous fluid indicates ischaemic bowel with severe enough damage to allow red blood cell leakage through the capillary wall. As the infarctive process progresses, an increase in white cell numbers results in the fluid becoming reddish brown and very turbid. For such changes to take place, the damaged intestine must be in direct contact with the peritoneal cavity. Horses with intussusception or bowel contained in the omental bursa or herniated into the chest may have normal peritoneal fluid. In generalized peritonitis the fluid is orange/yellow and opaque.

The early signs of almost all diseases are not associated with concurrent changes in peritoneal fluid. This is true of cases of strangulation obstruction where the lesion has not progressed enough for protein or cell leakage (i.e. during approximately the first 2 hours). Cases of peritonitis and non-strangulating infarction have peritoneal fluid changes at the time clinical signs are first observed. In horses with simple obstruction, a slow increase in the protein level of peritoneal fluid takes place with no concurrent rise in red or white blood cells. The neutrophil–macrophage ratio remains normal unless the obstruction causes ischaemia. A more dramatic increase in total protein in the fluid to more than 3 g/dl is seen in anterior enteritis. The absence of significant blood staining of fluid is of value in differentiating this syndrome from strangulating obstructions of the small

Table 11.3 Peritoneal fluid as a diagnostic aid.

	Colour	Turbidity	RBCs	Neutrophils	Protein	Bacteria
Normal	Pale yellow	Clear	None	$< 5000/\mu l$	$< 2.5\,g/dl$	None
Simple obstruction	Pale yellow	Clear	None	$< 5000/\mu l$	Slight increase	None
Early strangulation	Serosanguineous	Cloudy	Moderate numbers	Slight increase	Slight increase	None
Late strangulation	Red/brown	Opaque to flocculent	Moderate numbers	Marked neutrophilia	$> 3.5\,g/dl$	Some enteric
Anterior enteritis	Yellow	Clear	Usually none	Usually only slightly raised	$> 3.0\,g/dl$	None
Grass sickness	Yellow	Clear	None	Not raised	$> 3.0\,g/dl$	None
Septic peritonitis	Serosanguineous to purulent	Turbid to purulent	Variable	Often $> 100000/\mu l$	Raised	Sometimes present

RBC, red blood cells.

intestine, although if mural necrosis is advanced this distinction is not possible. In grass sickness the peritoneal fluid is clear but shows a similar increase in protein levels.

DISCUSSION

The diagnosis of primary gastric dilatation is usually straightforward, based on acute pain, stable systemic signs and the acid pH of the stomach contents. Evacuation of the stomach by nasogastric intubation is followed by immediate relief of pain and the resumption of normal borborygmi. Differentiating between the causes of secondary dilatation is not so simple. Palpation of distended small intestine in conjunction with gastric reflux almost always means that an obstruction has occurred which requires surgical correction. The disease that may not require surgical intervention is anterior enteritis, which may be suspected on the basis of gastric reflux associated with depression, fever, a neutrophilia, high protein levels in peritoneal fluid with low white cell numbers and total ileus; a positive diagnosis, however, is only possible at laparotomy or necropsy when the characteristic petechial and ecchymotic haemorrhages in the serosa of the proximal small intestine can be identified. Therefore, when any doubt exists about the diagnosis, exploratory laparotomy is fully justified. Any delay will risk progression of a strangulating lesion, if present, and a decreased chance of survival.

Various methods of treatment of anterior enteritis have been reported, both medical and surgical. Although it has been stated that the mortality rate increases substantially when horses with anterior enteritis undergo general anaesthesia and exploratory surgery (Blackwell, 1987), this has not been the author's experience. Prompt recourse to surgery, during which the distended small intestine was decompressed by gently stripping its contents into the caecum, together with intravenous metronidazole and fluid therapy, resulted in 23 of 24 horses making a rapid and uneventful recovery (Edwards, 1992).

In the UK, the existence of grass sickness further complicates the issue. The similarities between the presenting signs in this disease and anterior enteritis are obvious, namely colic and depression, gastric reflux, small intestinal distension, complete ileus and peritoneal fluid with a raised protein level and no white blood cells. Grass sickness is non-febrile and other signs such as muscular tremors, patchy sweating and salivation may help the diagnosis. However, these signs are often intermittent. Lateral radiography of the cervical and thoracic oesophagus following administration of barium sulphate has been used to identify the oesophageal dysfunction and dilatation which may be present (Greet and Whitwell, 1986). Plasma catecholamine levels have been shown to be higher than in normal horses or those with obstructive colic (Hodson et al., 1984).

However, these investigations entail the use of complex techniques which will not provide an instant diagnosis. Therefore, in the majority of cases, an exploratory laparotomy is performed to eliminate a physical obstruction and anterior enteritis. However, it is not uncommon to find secondary ileal impaction or malposition of the colon in horses with grass sickness. Until recently, there was no other option but to clear the impaction or correct the displacement and, having allowed the horse to recover from the anaesthesia, to await developments. The development of a diagnostic technique involving an ileal biopsy for evidence of specific intrinsic nerve damage (Scholes et al., 1993) now enables a diagnosis of grass sickness to be confirmed within 24 hours of the laparotomy. In view of the incurable nature of the condition, humane destruction is then carried out without delay.

ABDOMINAL CATASTROPHE

The possibility of gastric rupture having occurred in any horse suspected of having gastric dilatation should always be borne in mind, particularly if there is sudden cessation of overt signs of visceral pain followed by rapid progressive systemic deterioration. Retrieval of gas and no (or only a small volume of) fluid on passing a nasogastric tube in a horse which has been in colic for 12–24 hours and has numerous loops of distended small intestine palpable on rectal examination is highly suspicious. A peritoneal tap will reveal dark-brown fluid in which particles of food material can usually be identified. Further confirmation of this abdominal catastrophe is obtained when, on rectal examination, the serosal surfaces of the gut are felt to be rough owing to adherent particles of digesta, and free gas in the abdominal cavity makes it surprisingly easy to pass a hand between loops of distended small intestine.

A significant number of horses sent to referral centres are found on admission to have gastric rupture. While in some cases this may have happened in transit, in others it will have occurred before the horse was loaded. To avoid unnecessary suffering it is imperative that gastric rupture is diagnosed promptly and that the horse is euthanased immediately on humane grounds.

REFERENCES AND FURTHER READING

Bishop, A. E., Hodson, N. P., Major, J. H. *et al.* (1984) The regulatory peptide system of the large bowel in Equine Grass Sickness. *Experientia* **40**, 180–186.

Blackwell, R. B. (1987) Duodenitis in proximal enteritis. In *Current Therapy in Equine Medicine*, 2nd edn (ed. N. E. Robinson), pp. 44–45. W. B. Saunders, Philadelphia.

Edwards, G. B. (1992) Anterior enteritis as a surgical problem. *Proceedings of the North American Veterinary Conference*, Orlando, Florida, January, pp. 423–425.

Greet, T. R. C. & Whitwell, K. E. (1986) Radiological features of the equine oesophagus in grass sickness. *Equine Veterinary Journal* **18**, 294–297.

Hodson, N. P., Causon, R. & Edwards, G. B. (1984) Catecholamines in equine grass sickness. *Veterinary Record* **115**, 18–19.

Scholes, F. E. S., Vaillant, C., Peacock, P. J. & Edwards, G. B. (1993) Diagnosis of grass sickness by ileal biopsy. *Veterinary Record* **133** (1), 7–10.

Index